Clinical Pathology and Laboratory Techniques for Veterinary Technicians

Clinical Pathology and Laboratory Techniques for Veterinary Technicians

Edited by

Anne M. Barger, DVM, MS, Diplomate ACVP
Clinical Professor, Clinical Pathology, University of Illinois

Amy L. MacNeill, DVM, PhD, Diplomate ACVP
Associate Professor, Clinical Pathology, Colorado State University

WILEY Blackwell

This edition first published 2015 ©2015 by John Wiley & Sons, Inc

Editorial offices: 1606 Golden Aspen Drive, Suites 103 and 104, Ames, Iowa 50010, USA
The Atrium, Southern Gate, Chichester, West Sussex, PO19 8SQ, UK
9600 Garsington Road, Oxford, OX4 2DQ, UK

For details of our global editorial offices, for customer services and for information about how to apply for permission to reuse the copyright material in this book please see our website at www.wiley.com/wiley-blackwell.

Library of Congress Cataloging-in-Publication Data

Clinical pathology and laboratory techniques for veterinary technicians / edited by Anne M. Barger and Amy L. MacNeill.
      p. ; cm.
   Includes bibliographical references and index.
     ISBN 978-1-118-34509-2 (paperback)
1. Veterinary clinical pathology. I. Barger, Anne M., editor. II. MacNeill, Amy L., editor.
   [DNLM: 1. Clinical Laboratory Techniques–veterinary. 2. Animal Technicians. 3. Pathology, Clinical–methods. 4. Pathology, Veterinary–methods. SF 772.6]
   SF772.6.C55 2015
   636.089′607–dc23

                                                                                                         2015006610

A catalogue record for this book is available from the British Library.

Wiley also publishes its books in a variety of electronic formats. Some content that appears in print may not be available in electronic books.

Cover image: [Production Editor to insert]
Cover design by [Production Editor to insert]

Set in 10/12pt SabonLTStd by Laserwords Private Limited, Chennai, India

1   2015

Amy MacNeill Dedication:

This book is dedicated to Dr. Bruce Ferguson, who taught me many of the techniques in this text and nourished my love of veterinary medicine.

Anne Barger Dedication:

I would to thank my partner in life Dr. Patty McElroy and my father Maurice Barger for their continued love and support.

Contents

Chapter 6

Chapter 7

List of Contributors

Anne M. Barger
University of Illinois, Champaign, IL, USA

Bente Flatland
University of Tennessee, Knoxville, TN, USA

Amy L. MacNeill
Colorado State University, Fort Collins, CO, USA

Allan J. Paul
University of Illinois, Champaign, IL, USA

Amelia G. White
Auburn University, Auburn, AL, USA

Preface

The objective of this text is to provide a thorough, practical guide to clinical pathology. It is directed toward veterinary technician students, veterinary technicians in practice, and veterinarians in general practice. Included in this text are learning objectives for students and educators, many high-quality images of techniques, instrumentation, microscopic cells, organisms, and patients. Each chapter contains cases meant to allow the student to understand the practical application of the material.

About the Companion Website

This book is accompanied by a companion website:

www.wiley.com/go/barger/vettechclinpath

The website includes:

- Instructor questions
- Answers to the Multiple Choice Questions that are in the book
- Powerpoints of all figures from the book for downloading

The password for the site is the last word in the caption for Figure 2.11.

nucleus

Getting Started with Clinical Pathology

Amy L. MacNeill
Colorado State University, Fort Collins,
CO, USA

Learning Objectives

1. Become familiar with the equipment used to perform clinical pathology testing.
2. Understand when to use different types of blood collection tubes.
3. Know the sample types needed for clinical pathology tests.
4. Be able to process and store samples for clinical pathology tests.
5. Follow basic laboratory safety procedures.

KEY TERMS

Clinical pathology
Laboratory
Equipment
Supplies
Maintenance
Safety

Case example 1

A feline blood sample was collected into a blood tube containing EDTA, but the amount of blood in the tube was below the volume indicator on the side of the tube. The veterinary technician loaded the appropriate amount of the sample into the automated hematology analyzer. Results indicated that the cat had low erythrocyte and platelet counts. The technician recorded that the tube was underfilled before the results were reported. Why is it critical that the technician recorded the fact that the sample was underfilled?

Clinical Pathology and Laboratory Techniques for Veterinary Technicians, First Edition.
Edited by Anne Barger and Amy MacNeill.
© 2015 John Wiley & Sons, Inc. Published 2015 by John Wiley & Sons, Inc.
Companion Website: www.wiley.com/go/barger/vettechclinpath

Case example 2

A glass slide with dried blood on it was dropped on the floor and shattered. The animal caretaker saw the mess and began to pick up the pieces of glass with her bare hands. What should you do?

Introduction

Clinical pathology evaluates disease in animals using *laboratory* data collected during analysis of blood, urine, body fluids, and tissue aspirates. Laboratory data sets collected in sick animals typically include hematology data, serum or plasma chemistry concentrations, urinalysis results, and cytology interpretations. This chapter introduces the *equipment* used to collect accurate laboratory data.

Standard Equipment

A. Microscope.
   A well-maintained and properly aligned microscope is an important tool for analysis of blood smears, fecal samples, and urine sediment samples. This is an expensive tool that requires proper training to maximize the full potential use of the instrument.
   - Types of microscopes.
       There are several types of microscopes available (e.g., upright binocular light microscopes, inverted binocular fluorescent microscopes, and dissection monocular light microscopes). The most commonly used microscope in a veterinary clinic is an upright binocular light microscope. This type of microscope has a light source located below the sample stage, an objective lens located above the sample stage, and two eyepiece lenses that the user looks through simultaneously to visualize the sample. Figure 1.1 is a diagram of a typical upright binocular light microscope.
   - Components of an upright binocular light microscope.
       - Eyepieces typically hold lenses that magnify the sample by 10-fold (10×).
       - Draw tubes may or may not be present, depending on the brand of microscope. Draw tubes allow for minimal adjustment of sample focus to accommodate differences in visual acuity between each eye.
       - The body tube is the hollow section of the microscope between the eyepieces and the objective lenses.
       - The arm of the microscope supports the body tube and connects the eyepieces to the base of the microscope.
       - Objective lenses magnify the sample. The strength of magnification and whether or not the lens requires immersion oil to focus on the sample are

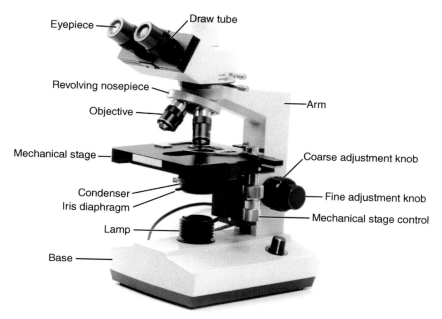

Figure 1.1   Microscope diagram. Components of an upright binocular light microscope are indicated. Common microscope components include two eyepieces, two draw tubes, a body tube, an arm, objective lenses, a revolving nosepiece, the microscope stage, stage clips, a mechanical stage control, a course adjustment knob, a fine adjustment knob, a condenser, an iris diaphragm, a lamp, and a rheostat. (*Source*: Adapted from Stock.com/David Ahn).

indicated on the side of the objective lens. For most clinical pathology tests performed in veterinary clinics, at least three objective lenses are recommended; a low power lens, a dry high power lens, and a high power lens that requires immersion oil for fine focusing.
- Objective lenses are attached to a revolving nosepiece so that the user can easily switch between objective lenses while looking at a sample. Properly aligned microscopes require very minimal movement of the fine adjustment knob to sharpen the focus between the different objective lenses.
- The microscope stage holds the sample under the objective lens and over the light source. A stage may have stage clips that secure the sample onto the stage if the microscope has a mechanical stage control.
- A mechanical stage control allows the user to move the sample around the stage via a joystick.
- A course adjustment knob allows the user to focus the sample using scanning and low-power lenses. This knob should not be adjusted when using high-power lenses.
- The fine adjustment knob is used to make subtle changes that bring the sample into fine, crisp focus when using high power lenses.
- A condenser is located between the bottom of the stage and the light source so that light scatter can be minimized.

- There is a condenser height adjustment knob in front of the coarse adjustment knob that changes the location of the condenser relative to the stage.
  - Condenser adjustment knobs are also located just below the condenser and are used to center the light source on the sample and align the light with the field of view through the eyepieces.
- An iris diaphragm is found over the light source of a microscope.
- The lamp of the microscope is the light source. Most microscopes have a rheostat located on the base that can be used to adjust the brightness of the light source.
- The microscope base should be placed on a clean, flat surface for proper use of the instrument.
- Magnification.
  - 2×, 4×, and 5× dry lenses are considered scanning lenses.
  - 10× and 20× dry lenses are examples of low power lenses.
  - 40× and 60× lenses are high power lenses that usually are dry lenses. A cover slip must be used with these objectives to prevent contaminating the lens with the sample.
  - 50× and 100× lenses are high power lenses that usually require immersion oil to allow the user to focus on the sample.
  - Most microscopes in veterinary practices have 10× and 40× dry lenses and a 100× oil lens.

> **TECHNICIAN TIP 1–1: TOTAL MAGNIFICATION**   The total magnification of a sample equals the product of the objective lens magnification and the magnification of the eyepiece lens. For example, if you are looking at a sample at "high power" (40× objective lens) and you have a 10× eyepiece lens, the total magnification of the sample is (40 × 10) = 400×.

- Specimen evaluation.
    Different sample types are prepared for microscopic examination in different ways. Whole blood typically is smeared onto a glass slide, dried, and stained before examination. Urine sediment, on the other hand, is examined as a wet mount after the sample has been centrifuged, concentrated, resuspended in a smaller volume of urine, dropped onto a slide, and then covered with a cover slip. Feces can be examined as a direct smear after being stained or as a wet mount after fecal flotation has been performed. These processes are described in detail in other chapters of this book. The focus of this section is to describe how to examine dry, stained smears, and wet mounts using a microscope.
  - The microscope needs to be on a flat surface near access to an electrical power outlet to plug in the light source.
  - Microscope lenses should be properly installed and clean.
  - Typically, the iris is kept opened when examining a sample for clinical pathology tests but may be closed slightly to reduce the amount of light reaching the sample or to minimize light scatter, if needed.

- Samples must be thin enough to allow light to shine through the specimen.
- A scanning objective lens or 10× low power lens should be in place, aimed toward the microscope stage.
- A glass microscope slide containing the sample is placed onto the microscope stage carefully. This often requires fitting the slide between stage clips.
  - To examine dry, stained smears, the condenser is raised up, close to the stage (Figure 1.2a).
  - To examine a wet mount, the condenser should be lowered down, away from the stage (Figure 1.2b).
- Look into the eyepieces, turn on the light source, and adjust the light using the rheostat so that it is not painful to the eyes. Focus on the sample using a scanning or 10× lens and the coarse adjustment knob. If draw tubes are present, the focus can be adjusted individually to each eye.
- Switch to a dry high power objective lens by moving the revolving nosepiece to the proper position. Make small adjustments to the focus using the fine adjustment knob. Complete any analysis you can while focused on the sample with the dry objective lens.
  - The 40× objective lens is the highest magnification used for wet mounts.
  - DO NOT use the course adjustment knob to focus on the slide using a high power objective lens; it is highly likely that the slide will crack or the lens will be damaged.
- If the sample is a dry, stained smear, place a small drop of immersion oil onto the sample and use the revolving nosepiece to move the high power oil lens in place for final data collection.
- NOTE: You cannot switch back to a dry objective lens once oil has been placed on the sample.

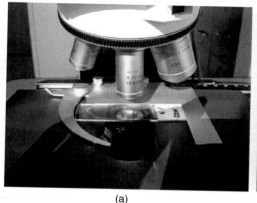 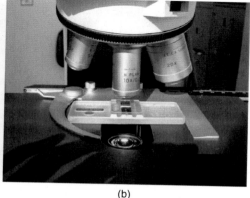

(a)   (b)

Figure 1.2   Microscope condenser settings. (a) Dried samples are examined with the condenser close to the microscope stage to reduce light scatter. (b) Fluid samples (including wet-mounted samples and hemocytometers) are examined with the condenser lowered away from the microscope stage to improve visualization of objects that are floating in solution.

TECHNICIAN TIP 1–2: WAYS TO FIX COMMON PROBLEMS WITH THE MICROSCOPE

- The viewing field is too dark.
    - Open the iris diaphragm.
    - Increase the light intensity.
    - Be sure that the condenser is up near the slide if the sample is a dry, stained smear.
- There is a stationary spot in the field of view that does not move when the slide is moved.
    - Use lens cleaning solution and lens paper to clean the eyepieces.
    - Use lens cleaning solution and lens paper to clean the objective lens.
    - Remove the eyepieces and clean any debris at the bottom of the draw tube with lens paper.
    - Wipe off the condenser with lens paper.
    - Wipe off the light source with lens paper.
- The view field is cloudy or cannot be perfectly focused using the 40× objective lens.
    - Use lens cleaning solution and lens paper to clean the objective lens.
    - Place a coverslip on the slide to improve the performance of the 40× lens.
        - A coverslip can be placed onto a slide using immersion oil or mounting medium.
- The view field is partially lit and partially black.
    - Check the positioning of the objective lens.
    - Be sure that the light is centered on the sample (see Microscope maintenance).

- Microscope maintenance.
    Microscopes should be serviced at least once a year by a professional microscopist. Daily maintenance must be performed by clinic staff.
    - Daily maintenance includes the following:
        - Keeping the lenses, condenser, and light source clean of debris using lens cleaning solution and lens paper. Avoid scratching the surface of the lenses.
        - Centering the light on the sample.
            - Set the scanning lens in place using the revolving nosepiece.
            - Close the iris diaphragm.
            - Lower the condenser. A small spot of light should be visible in the field of view.
            - Center the spot of light using the condenser adjustment knobs.
            - Raise the condenser.
            - Open the iris diaphragm.
    - To safely move a microscope, hold onto the arm of the microscope with one hand and support the base of the microscope with the other hand.
    - DO NOT get oil on a dry lens. If oil does get on a dry lens, it will need to be carefully and thoroughly cleaned using lens cleaning solution and lens paper.
    - Be sure to turn off the light source and cover the microscope with a plastic bag or microscope cover after use.
B. Centrifuge.
    Working centrifuges are needed to process samples for clinical pathology testing. It is imperative that centrifuges are used correctly and cleaned routinely to avoid

damage to the machine. To clean a centrifuge, wipe all surfaces with dilute soapy water, rinse with water, and allow the parts to dry completely before using the centrifuge. Do not use metal brushes or sharp objects to remove debris from rotors or sample holder; if these components are scratched, they will need to be replaced.

Centrifuges are designed to spin a rotor, which holds the samples, at a specific set speed measured in revolutions per minute (rpm). The length of the rotor arm varies in different centrifuges. The length of the rotor arm and speed of the spin determine the gravitational force (g) that a sample is subjected to. The g force causes larger, heavier components of the sample to gravitate to the bottom of the sample tube and lighter, less dense components to remain at the top of the sample. For example, in a blood sample, cells will pellet at the bottom of a centrifuged tube and lipids will remain near the top of the sample.

Centrifuge rotors should be examined yearly for pitting or warping of the metal. Damaged rotors are not safe to use and need to be replaced. There are two common types of rotors, fixed rotors and swinging bucket rotors. An example of a fixed rotor is found in a microhematocrit centrifuge. In a swinging bucket rotor, all buckets *always* should be placed into the rotor before using the machine to avoid warping the rotor. Either type of rotor must have a balanced load before the centrifuge is turned on. This means if a sample is placed in one sample holder, an equal weight must be put in the sample holder located directly across from the sample (Figure 1.3).

C. Refractometer.

Refractometry is an analytical method that correlates the degree of light refraction (refractive index) in a liquid with the amount of solids in the liquid. Refractometers are available in most veterinary practices and commonly are used to determine protein concentration and specific gravity of fluid samples.

To use a refractometer, lift the clear lid and fill the refractometer with the liquid (Figure 4.10d). Close the clear lid and angle the refractometer toward a light (Figure 4.10e). Look through the eyepiece of the refractometer and locate the scale (Figure 1.4). Adjust the eyepiece by turning it back and forth to bring the scale into focus. Read the scale with the appropriate units for the solid or property you are measuring. For example, the units for the total protein of a sample are grams per deciliter. Because this technique relies on light to be able to pass through the liquid, both hemolysis and lipemia can interfere with accuracy.

D. Hemocytometer.

A hemocytometer is a specialized chamber with a small precise grid used to perform manual cell counts when cells are suspended in a liquid medium (Figure 1.5a). A specific type of coverslip must be used with the hemocytometer to ensure that the proper volume of fluid is loaded onto the chamber; otherwise, cell counts will be inaccurate.

- Using a hemocytometer.
  - Before using a hemocytometer, be sure that the hemocytometer and coverslip are clean.
  - Place the coverslip onto the chamber.
  - Add 10 µL of well-mixed sample fluid onto each side of the hemocytometer (Figure 1.5b).

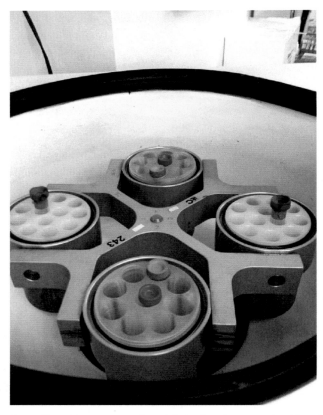

Figure 1.3   Balanced centrifuge. The same sample weight is placed on opposite sides of a centrifuge rotor to balance the sample load during centrifugation. This prevents damage to the rotor.

- Allow the cells to settle by incubating the hemocytometer for 10 minutes in a petri dish containing a wet piece of absorbent paper (Figure 1.5c).
- Using the microscope with the condenser lowered (Figure 1.2b), determine the average number of cells present in 1-mm grid section on the hemocytometer (Figure 1.6).
- The average number of cells in one 1-mm grid is the number of cells per 0.1 μL of sample fluid. The following bullet points give an example of how to use a hemocytometer to calculate the number of cells per microliter of sample fluid.
  - NOTE: There are nine 1-mm grid sections on each chamber of the hemocytometer.
    - Cells in the middle of a 1-mm grid and touching the top and left edges of a 1-mm grid should be counted.
    - Do not count cells touching the bottom and right edges of a 1-mm grid.

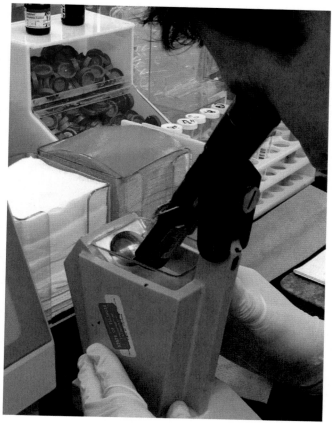

Figure 1.4   Refractometer measurement. The proportion of solids in a fluid sample is calculated by a refractometer. This value is read by looking through the eyepiece of the instrument and adjusting the eyepiece to fine focus the scale present in the refractometer.

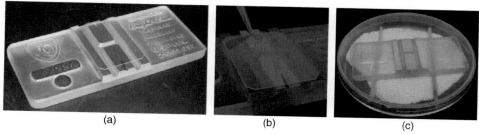

(a)   (b)   (c)

Figure 1.5   Hemocytometer. (a) Hemocytometer with two chambers for counting the number of cells in a fluid sample. (b) Ten microliters of fluid is loaded into each chamber of a hemocytometer. (c) Hemocytometer incubating in a petri dish over a damp gauze to prevent the sample from drying out and allow the cells to settle.

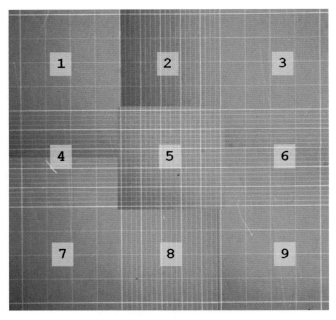

Figure 1.6   Hemocytometer grid. Each chamber of a hemocytometer contains nine 1-mm grid sections. Cells that fall within the grid section and on the upper and left edges of the grid section are counted. Cells that fall on the lower and right edges of the grid section are not counted.

- At least five 1-mm grid sections from each side of the hemocytometer should be counted to determine the average number of cells/grid.
- Ideally, the variation between cell counts from the two chambers of the hemocytometer should not exceed 10%.
- Calculate cells/µL using the formula:
  - (Cells/grid × sample dilution) ÷ 0.1 µL/grid = cells/µL
  - Example: If the sample dilution factor is 1:2000 and the average number of cells in one grid section is 200, then (200 cells/grid × 2000) ÷ 0.1 µL/grid = 4×10^6 cells/µL.

E. Differential cell counter.

A differential cell counter allows as user to keep track of the cell types observed and the total number of cells examined on a sample slide. Both analog (Figure 1.7a) and digital (Figure 1.7b) differential cell counters are available. Different buttons on the cell counter are assigned to different cell types. When a particular cell type is identified microscopically, the user presses a button assigned to that cell type. Each time the button is pressed, the number recorded on the instrument increases by one. Different numbers are recorded for each button representing each cell type identified. Simultaneously, the total number of cells examined is tallied and recorded. The counters are set to indicate when 100 cells are tallied.

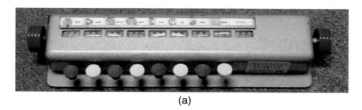

(a)

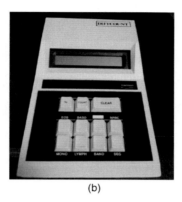

(b)

Figure 1.7   Differential cell counters. (a) Analog and (b) digital cell counters are shown.

Standard Supplies

A. Stain.
  - Cells are more easily identified if they have been stained with dyes. For blood smears and cytology samples, Romanowski-type stains are used most commonly.
  - Samples are thinly smeared onto a glass microscope slide so that they are arranged in a single-cell layer. Then the slides are allowed to dry before they are exposed to cellular dyes.
  - There are several types of stains available for microscopic examination of cells. The most common stains used in veterinary practices are Romanowski-type stains and new methylene blue (NMB) stain.
    - Often, cells stained using Romanowski-types stains are fixed in methanol before staining with a cationic dye and an anionic dye. This fixation step allows the dyes to enter the cell membrane and bind intracellular structures.
      - The cationic dye stains acidic cell structures (such as nuclear material and acidic proteins) a blue–purple color.
      - Basic cell structures, including most cellular proteins, bind the anionic dye and stain red.
      - Romanowski-type stains include Diff-Quik®, Wright–Giemsa, May–Grunwald–Giemsa, and Leishman's stains.

- Diff-Quik® staining procedure.
  - Repeatedly dip a dried sample that has been thinly smeared onto a glass slide in and out of the first staining solution 10–12 times.
    - This solution is clear or light blue.
    - Methanol can be used for this step.
  - Repeatedly dip the sample in and out of the second staining solution ten times.
    - This solution is red.
  - Repeatedly dip the sample in and out of the third staining solution eight to ten times.
    - This solution is blue.
  - Rinse the slide in deionized water to remove excess stain. Tap water can be used if deionized water is unavailable but staining characteristics may be slightly altered.
  - Allow the slide to air dry and then examine the sample microscopically.
- NMB staining procedure. This stain dyes acidic groups (including DNA and RNA) blue. Primarily, NMB is used to detect immature red blood cells (RBCs) and oxidative damage to RBCs.
  - Mix equal amounts of NMB and blood (or other fluid sample) together in a test tube.
  - Incubate for 5–10 minutes.
  - Prepare a smear of the NMB/sample mixture and allow it to air dry.
  - Examine the smear microscopically.

B. Glass slides.

Glass slides used for microscopy need to be precleaned before packaging to avoid glass shards and greasy substances that accumulate on the slide during the manufacturing process. Vendors that sell glass slides will specify if the slides have been precleaned.

All samples, including glass slides, should be labeled well enough to identify the patient that the sample was collected from, the date of collection, and type of sample. Glass slides should be labeled using a pencil, a marker specifically designated for sample labeling, or a glass etching tool. Otherwise, the label is likely to wash off when the sample is stained. Slides may come with or without a frosted edge. The frosted edge is convenient for labeling the sample. However, if part of the sample is accidentally smeared over the frosted edge, that part of the sample cannot be visualized under the microscope and diagnostic material may be lost.

> **TECHNICIAN TIP 1–3: LABELING SLIDES**　Ink pen and marker will wash off of glass slides when samples are stained. When labeling slides, use a pencil, a marker specifically designated for sample labeling, or a glass etching tool.

C. Coverslips.

Coverslips are needed for wet-mount preparations of fluid samples. In addition, coverslips should be placed over all samples dried onto glass slides to allow for crisp focusing of the microscope when using a high power objective lens. Coverslips may be placed onto a sample using immersion oil or specialized glue (mounting medium). When glued on, coverslips can preserve samples for a long period of time.

D. Blood tubes.

There are several types of tubes that are used for collection of blood. Specific types of tubes are needed for different types of clinical pathology tests. Avoid positive pressure when filling tubes, forcing the blood into the tube by pressing on the syringe can result in hemolysis. Let the tube fill via vacuum pressure or remove the rubber stopper on the tube to break the vacuum. Tubes should be filled with the appropriate amount of blood as indicated on the side of the tube. This will ensure that the tube contains the correct ratio of the chemical in the tube and the blood.

- Types of blood collection tubes (Figure 1.8) and their uses:
  - Striped-red- and gray-topped tubes
    - Used to collect serum
    - Also known as serum separator tubes

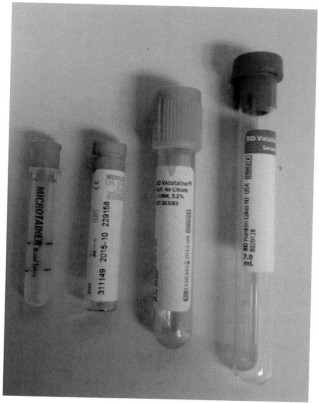

Figure 1.8   Blood collection tubes. Different blood collection tubes are needed for different clinical pathology diagnostic tests. These tubes come in many different sizes and are color coded for easy identification.

- As the clotted sample is centrifuged, a gel moves between the clot and the serum to prevent alterations in serum chemistry values.
- Serum separator tubes should not be used for samples drawn to measure drug concentrations because contact with the serum separator gel may falsely decrease results.
- Red-topped tubes
  - Used to collect serum
  - Does NOT contain anticoagulant or serum separator gel
  - Once the sample has clotted, it needs to be centrifuged. Immediately after centrifugation, the serum must be removed from the blood clot and placed in a separate tube to avoid alterations in serum chemistry values.
- Purple-topped tubes
  - Used to collect whole blood
  - Contains the anticoagulant ethylenediaminetetraacetic acid (EDTA)
    - The final concentration of EDTA should be 1.8 mg/mL of blood.
  - Preferred collection tube for complete blood counts (CBCs) in mammals
- Green-topped tubes
  - Used to collect plasma
  - Contains the anticoagulant lithium heparin
    - The final concentration of heparin should be approximately 16 international units per milliliter of blood.
  - The sample can be centrifuged immediately (as the sample will not clot). After centrifugation, the plasma should be removed from the RBCs with a pipette and placed into another tube.
  - When submitting heparinized samples to an outside laboratory, label the sample as heparinized plasma so the laboratory knows what they are dealing with.
- Blue-topped tubes
  - Contain 3.2% sodium citrate
  - Dilutes the blood sample by 10%
  - Preferred for most platelet function tests

Sample Types

There are several sample types that may be submitted for analysis using clinical pathology tests. Below is a short list of the most common samples processed. These are the sample types discussed in this book.

A. Whole blood includes the unclotted cells and the fluid portion of the blood.
B. Serum is the fluid portion of the blood that remains after the formation of a blood clot.
C. Plasma is the fluid portion of the blood that remains after unclotted cells have been removed from the sample.
D. Urine is the fluid waste product removed from the blood by the kidneys.
E. Feces are solid waste products produced by the digestive tract.

Sample Storage and Preparation

The way that samples are manipulated in the laboratory has a direct effect on the accuracy of test results. The chapters in this book provide guidelines for storage and preparation of samples for several types of clinical pathology tests. If you are asked to process a sample for a test you are not familiar with, it is best to research the proper way to handle the sample before sample collection. If the sample is being shipped to another laboratory, speak with a customer service representative to ensure that the sample is collected, stored, and shipped properly. This will provide veterinarians with more reliable data, which should be a priority whenever a sample is processed for clinical pathology testing.

Basic Laboratory Safety

Every laboratory should designate a person to oversee the safety of the laboratory. Individuals that work in the laboratory must follow the safety guidelines that are in place. Some basic laboratory safety guidelines are listed in the following text:

A. Sharps.
   - Needles are encountered commonly in a laboratory setting. Sharps containers for proper disposal of needles should be easily accessible at all times. These containers must be closed, sealed, and removed from the laboratory before they become filled to the brim. Most containers have a fill line that should be observed.
   - Glass slides and tubes may break in the laboratory. If samples contain biologic materials, the glass should be cleaned up using a broom and a dust pan and then disposed of in a sharps container. If the glass does not contain sample material, it may be cleaned up using a broom and a dust pan and then disposed of in a trash container. Just be sure that the glass cannot break through the trash container and injure other workers.
B. Chemicals.
   Laboratories often store chemicals and solutions that are used in various tests. Material safety data sheets should be posted for each chemical. Familiarize yourself with this information so that spills or inadvertent contact with the material can be cleaned up and treated appropriately.
C. Biological materials.
   Clinical pathology laboratories process several types of potentially biohazardous materials including blood and feces. These samples must be handled properly to prevent alteration of the sample with environmental contaminants and to prevent contamination of the environment with infectious organisms from the samples. If samples are spilled, be sure to wear gloves when cleaning them up.
   - To clean a contaminated surface, soak the area in 10% bleach solution for at least 10 minutes and then wipe the area dry with disposable towels. Dispose of the towels into a garbage can.

- To clean contaminated clothing, remove soiled articles of clothing and wash them on site in 10% bleach solution. Do NOT bring contaminated clothing home to be laundered.

  Once processed, samples should be stored or disposed of. Typically, body fluids and feces are discarded into biohazard bags that are clearly marked with a biohazard symbol. These bags are then autoclaved before being placed into a proper garbage container.

D. Personal protective equipment (PPE).

  Personal protective equipment (PPE) includes gloves, laboratory coats, eye protection, masks, surgical caps, closed-toed shoes, and booties. Laboratories often require personnel to wear one or more of these items, particularly if potentially biohazardous samples are being processed in the laboratory. Gloves, laboratory coats, and closed-toed shoes are particularly important to minimize contamination of skin and clothing. Remember that gloves and laboratory coats should be removed as you are leaving the laboratory to avoid spreading any contaminants throughout the hospital. Always follow the PPE guidelines that are recommended by the laboratory you are working in.

Interpretation and comments for Case 1

It is important because the findings of anemia and thrombocytopenia may be inaccurate. The cell counts were likely decreased due to dilution of the sample by the EDTA in the tube.

Interpretation and comments for Case 2

Ask the caretaker to stop and wait until you get a broom and dustpan to clean up the glass. The glass can then be placed into a trash container. Be sure that the shards of glass do not protrude from the trash bag.

Activities

Multiple Choice Questions

1. Which component of the microscope should be adjusted when evaluating a wet-mount slide?
   A) 10× objective
   B) Stage
   C) Condenser
   D) Eyepiece

2. Where is the iris diaphragm located?
   A) In the eyepiece
   B) Above the stage
   C) Above the light source
   D) In the base

3. Which of the following are low power objective lenses?
   A) 4×
   B) 20×
   C) 40×
   D) 100×

4. Which objective lens requires immersion oil?
   A) 4×
   B) 20×
   C) 40×
   D) 100×

5. True/False: Swinging bucket centrifuges do not need to be balanced.

6. In a centrifuge, _____ and _____ determine the gravitational force that a sample is subjected.

7. Refractive index is:
   A) The degree of light refraction through a liquid.
   B) The optical density of water.
   C) Not dependent on the amount of solid in a liquid.
   D) Calculated from the density of the liquid.

8. Which tube is the preferred blood tube for CBCs in mammals?
   A) Serum separator tube (striped-red and gray topped tube)
   B) Heparin tube (green topped tube)
   C) EDTA tube (lavender topped tube)
   D) Serum tube (red topped tube)

Hematology

chapter 2

Amy L. MacNeill
Colorado State University, Fort Collins, CO,
USA

Learning Objectives

1. Become familiar with blood cell maturation and development (hematopoiesis).
2. Understand erythrocyte, leukocyte, and platelet functions.
3. Learn the medical terminology and abbreviations associated with hematologic parameters.
4. Identify changes in erythrocyte, leukocyte, and platelet morphology.
5. Identify inclusions within blood cells.
6. Determine erythrocyte, leukocyte, and platelet counts.
7. Perform a white blood cell differential count.
8. Describe abnormalities on a complete blood cell profile.
9. Follow common procedures used to diagnose diseases associated with hematologic abnormalities.

KEY TERMS

Basophil
Complete blood count
Eosinophil
Erythrocyte
Hemoglobin
Hematocrit
Leukocyte
Lymphocyte
Monocyte
Neutrophil
Platelet

Clinical Pathology and Laboratory Techniques for Veterinary Technicians, First Edition.
Edited by Anne Barger and Amy MacNeill.
© 2015 John Wiley & Sons, Inc. Published 2015 by John Wiley & Sons, Inc.
Companion Website: www.wiley.com/go/barger/vettechclinpath

Case example 1

Signalment: 10-year-old, intact, female, mixed-breed dog. History: Mammary gland adeno-
carcinoma diagnosed 1 year ago. Has had two radical mastectomies. Physical examination:
clinically dehydrated; pale, yellow and tacky mucous membranes. Plan: Blood was drawn
and placed into a purple-topped tube to collect whole blood for a CBC.

CBC

Parameter	Result	Reference Range
Hct	15%	35.0–57.0
Hgb	4.5 g/dL	11.9–18.9
RBC	$3.3 \times 10^6/\mu L$	$4.95–7.87 \times 10^6$
MCV	78 fL	60.0–77.0
MCHC	30 g/dL	32.0–36.3
Reticulocytes (uncorrected)	4.5%	
WBC	17,700/μL	6,000–17,000
Segmented neutrophils	15,753/μL	3,000– 11,500
Lymphocytes	531/μL	1,000–4,800
Monocytes	1,416/μL	150–1,350
Eosinophils	0/μL	100–1,250
Basophils	0/μL	0–100
Platelets	48,000/μL	200,000–600,000
RBC morphology	1+ spherocytes	

Case example 2

Signalment: 6-year-old, mare, quarter horse. History: 2-month history of diarrhea. Physical
examination: tacky mucous membranes, fever of 103°F. Plan: Blood was drawn and placed
into a green-topped tube to obtain a CBC and into a blue-topped tube to determine the
fibrinogen concentration.

CBC

Parameter	Result	Reference Range
PCV	55%	30–46
Hgb	18.4 g/dL	10–16
MCV	39 fL	37–53
MCHC	36 g/dL	34–38
WBC	15,500/μL	5,500–12,500
Segmented neutrophils	11,500/μL	2700-6700
Band neutrophils	1,000/μL	0–100
Monocytes	800/μL	0–800
Lymphocytes	2,200/μL	2500–7500
Eosinophils	0.0/μL	0–2,400
Platelets	400,000/μL	100,000–600,000
Fibrinogen	900 mg/dL	200–500

Case example 3

Signalment: 4-year-old, milking, Shorthorn cow. History and physical examination: down, pale mucous membranes. Plan: Blood was drawn and placed into a purple-topped tube to collect whole blood for a CBC.

CBC

Parameter	Result	Reference Range
Hct	23.4%	27.0–35.0
Hgb	7.8 g/dL	9.0–12.0
RBC	$4.80 \times 10^6/\mu L$	$5.00–7.00 \times 10^6$
MCV	48.7 fL	44.0–54.0
MCH	16.2 pg	14.0–20.0
MCHC	33.3 g/dL	33.0–35.0
RBC morphology	3+ echinocytes	
	1+ keratocytes	
WBC	$5.47 \times 10^3/\mu L$	4,000–10,000
Segmented neutrophils	1,620/μL	2,500–5,500
Band neutrophils	130/μL	0–100
Lymphocytes	3,000/μL	2,000–4,600
Monocytes	700/μL	200–800
Eosinophils	20/μL	0–400
Basophils	0/μL	0–100
Platelets	240,000/μL	200,000–700,000

Introduction

Hematology is the study of blood. Blood is composed of plasma and cells (erythrocytes, leukocytes, and platelets). A *complete blood count* (CBC) is a diagnostic test panel that provides clinicians with a large amount of information about a patient's peripheral blood parameters. Data reported in a CBC include the identity of cell types in the peripheral blood, the number of blood cells in a microliter of blood, information about blood cell maturation, and abnormalities in the morphology (microscopic appearance) of the cells. Additional measurements that often are reported with a CBC include packed cell volume (PCV), plasma protein concentration, and fibrinogen concentration.

CBCs are routinely performed in sick patients because abnormalities present in the peripheral blood can indicate what type of disease process is occurring in the patient. Therefore, identification of abnormalities in blood cells is one of the most important skills for a veterinary technician to have. This chapter describes the functions of blood, depicts abnormalities found in blood cells, and outlines methods for obtaining a CBC and performing additional hematologic tests.

Components of Peripheral Blood

A. Plasma

   In health, plasma comprises approximately 55% of the total blood volume. Plasma is isolated by collecting blood in an anticoagulant (ethylenediaminetetraacetic acid [EDTA], heparin, or citrate) and centrifuging the sample to pellet out the cells. When blood is collected without an anticoagulant and allowed to clot before it is centrifuged, the supernatant fluid is called serum. Serum contains most of the elements in plasma except for some clotting factors and fibrinogen (which are consumed during clot formation).
   - Plasma is made up of
     - 91.5% water
     - 7% plasma proteins
       - Albumin, globulins, and fibrinogen
     - 1.5% other molecules
       - Salts, lipids, hormones, vitamins, and carbohydrates
   - Plasma has several important functions:
     - Transportation of cells and nutrients throughout the body
     - Excretion of by-products and waste
     - Maintenance of homeostasis via stabilization of pH and body temperature
   - Plasma from cats and dogs should be clear and colorless. Plasma from horses is clear and light yellow because they tend to have higher bilirubin concentrations than other species. Plasma from cattle is clear and colorless or pale yellow because of their herbivorous diets.

B. Blood cells

   Cells (*erythrocytes*, *leukocytes*, and *platelets)* comprise approximately 45% of the total blood volume.
   - Blood cells have a limited life span and are continually being produced by a process called hematopoiesis. Hematopoiesis occurs in the bone marrow (medullary hematopoiesis) and in several organs (extramedullary hematopoiesis). During hematopoiesis, blood cells develop from immature, blast cells to fully functional, mature cells that are released into the peripheral blood so that they can circulate throughout the body.
   - During hematopoiesis, cellular appearance (morphology) changes. The different stages of cell maturation can be identified microscopically if the cells are stained properly. The most common types of cellular stains that are used are Romanowski-type stains (see Chapter 1). Morphological differences in blood cell types are emphasized later in this chapter.

Blood Cell Parameters

- The most common way to acquire blood cell parameters is by using an automated hematology analyzer. When whole blood has been processed properly and the analyzer has been calibrated for the appropriate species, automated instruments are good to excellent at reporting accurate erythrocyte and leukocyte counts as well as erythrocyte and platelet indices. They are good at reporting platelet counts if there are no platelet clumps in the sample. Nearly all automated analyzers are poor to fair at reporting accurate leukocyte differential counts (particularly if the patient sample contains basophils). None of the automated analyzers adequately report changes in cellular morphology. For these reasons, hematology analyzers are valuable tools, but they are insufficient for producing a full CBC. A blood smear must be examined by a competent technician or veterinarian.

- There are two types of automated hematology analyzers, impedance counters and flow cytometers.
  - Impedance counters measure the electrical impedance that occurs when cells pass through detection electrodes. The change in voltage that occurs corresponds to the size and type of the cell that passes through the analyzer.
  - Flow cytometers direct cells through the path of a laser beam. They detect the amount of light absorbed by the cell and the amount of light scatter that the cell creates as it passes through. This allows the machine to determine cell size and complexity. In some analyzers, additional reagents and channels can be added to differentiate WBC subtypes, determine reticulocyte counts, and identify immature platelets (reticulated platelets). Specialized erythrocyte and platelet indices can also be reported by some analyzers.
- The most current analyzers available incorporate flow cytometry to determine cell type and indices.
- Examples of hematology analyzers that are commonly used in the veterinary clinical setting include
  - ProCyte Dx™ Hematology Analyzer from IDEXX
  - HemaTrue Hematology Analyzer from Heska
  - XT-2000iV Automated Hematology Analyzer from Sysmex
- Examples of hematology analyzers that are commonly used in veterinary diagnostic laboratories include
  - CELL-DYN 3700 from Abbott
  - ADVIA® 120 from Siemens
  - XS-Series from Sysmex
- Quality control is extremely important to ensure that accurate data is being reported by an instrument.
  - The precision and accuracy of a hematology analyzer should be evaluated frequently.
  - Reference intervals for each species must be established for each instrument at each location.
  - Refer to guidelines presented in Chapter 7 for more information on quality control and instrument validation.

Erythrocytes

A. Erythrocyte maturation
- Red blood cells are the predominant cell type in the peripheral blood.
- They originate in the bone marrow (and other sites of hematopoiesis) where they mature until they are released into the peripheral blood.
- The process of erythrocyte maturation is called erythropoiesis.
  - Cell size decreases during RBC maturation.
    - Mature RBCs have a lower mean cell volume (MCV) parameter than immature RBCs.
- Adequate erythropoiesis requires production of erythropoietin (EPO).
  - Most EPO is produced by renal tubular epithelial cells. Kidney disease may prevent adequate production of EPO that can lead to abnormally low numbers of RBCs in the peripheral blood.
  - Excess production of EPO is rare but may occur with some neoplastic diseases. Excess levels of EPO may cause a patient to have abnormally high numbers of RBCs in the peripheral blood.
- As erythrocytes mature, the cells become smaller, the cytoplasm stains less blue (basophilic) and more red (eosinophilic) with Romanowski-type stains, and the nucleus condenses.
  - Rubriblasts are the first identifiable immature form of an RBC. These cells are relatively large and have scant, deeply basophilic cytoplasm, a round nucleus, and a prominent nucleolus (Figure 2.1a).
    - Abnormal release of rubriblasts into the peripheral blood is extremely rare but can occur with acute erythroid leukemia.
  - Rubricytes are more mature and slightly smaller than rubriblasts but are larger and less mature than metarubricytes. Their cytoplasm is slightly less basophilic than a rubriblast and they have a round nucleus, but they lack a nucleolus (Figure 2.1b).
  - Metarubricytes also are called nucleated red blood cells (nRBCs). These cells are more mature and smaller than rubricytes. Metarubricytes are similar in size to reticulocytes which are only slightly larger than mature erythrocytes. They have polychromatophilic cytoplasm (meaning the cytoplasm simultaneously stains with basophilic and eosinophilic dyes). nRBCs contain a small, very condensed nucleus (Figure 2.1c).
    - nRBCs can be released into the peripheral blood when an animal is anemic (has a low RBC count) or is hypoxic (has low levels of oxygen in the peripheral blood).
    - Inappropriate release of nRBCs is associated with various splenic and bone marrow diseases as well as with lead toxicity, iron deficiency, and copper deficiency.
  - Reticulocytes are just slightly larger and slightly more basophilic than mature RBCs (Figures 2.1d and 2.2a). Owing to the combination of blue and red staining in these cells, they commonly are called polychromatophils.
    - Reticulocytes are expected to be released into the peripheral blood when an animal is anemic or hypoxic.

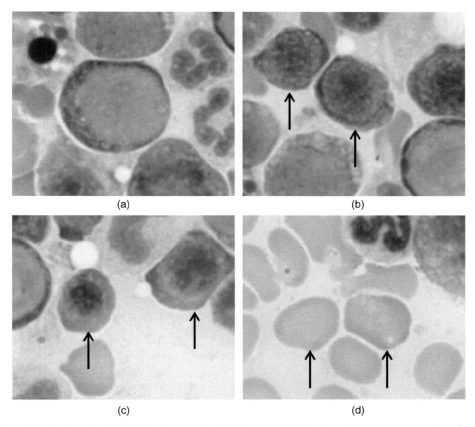

Figure 2.1   Erythropoiesis (Wright–Giemsa stain, 1400× magnification). (a–d) Bone marrow aspirate from a Bernese mountain dog. (a) Rubriblast with scant, deeply basophilic cytoplasm; a large, round nucleus; and three prominent nucleoli. (b) Rubricytes (arrows) with basophilic cytoplasm and a round nucleus with a clumped chromatin pattern. (c) Metarubricytes (arrows) with polychromatophilic cytoplasm and a small, condensed nucleus. (d) Reticulocytes (arrows) with polychromatophilic cytoplasm and no nucleus.

- Early release of reticulocytes into the peripheral blood does not occur in the horse.
- An increased reticulocyte count (reticulocytosis) indicates that the bone marrow is able to increase erythrocyte production in response to the body's demand for more erythrocytes to deliver oxygen (O_2) to the tissues. In other words, the bone marrow is regenerating erythrocytes appropriately.
- An anemic patient with an increased number of reticulocytes in the peripheral blood has a regenerative anemia.
- Patients that have been anemic for several days, but still do not have increased numbers of circulating reticulocytes, have a non-regenerative anemia.

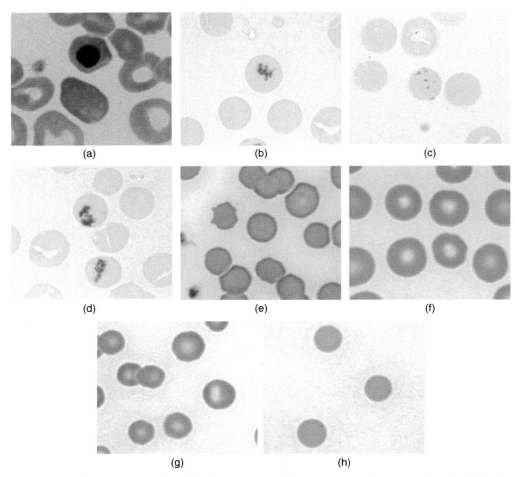

Figure 2.2 Erythrocytes in peripheral blood (1400× magnification). (a) Metarubricyte (nucleated red blood cell) from a Lhasa apso (Wright–Giemsa stain). (b-d) Blood from a Lhasa apso, new methylene blue stain. (b) Reticulocyte containing blue-staining RNA and ribosomes. (c) Punctate reticulocyte with small-rounded basophilic-staining remnants of RNA and ribosomes. (d) Aggregate reticulocytes with large clusters of basophilic-staining remnants of RNA and ribosomes. (e-h) Wright–Giemsa stain. (e) Erythrocytes from a domestic shorthaired cat. (f) Erythrocytes from a cocker spaniel showing central pallor. (g) Erythrocytes from a foal. (h) Bovine erythrocytes.

- This does not apply to horses.
- Non-regenerative anemia may be a poor prognostic indicator that can warrant bone marrow cytology and histopathology.
- Not all reticulocytes are polychromatophilic when stained with Romanowski-type stains. For this reason, reticulocyte counts are performed using new methylene blue (NMB) stain.
  - If Romanowski-type stains are used, polychromasia is scored as 1+, 2+, 3+, or 4+ and varies between species (Table 2.1).

Table 2.1   Polychromasia scoring system. Note that polychromasia will not be observed in the horse.

Polychromasia Score	Average Number of Polychromatophils/1000×	
	Cat & Cow	Dog
1+	0–1	1–2
2+	1–2	2–3
3+	2–4	3–6
4+	4+	6+

- Using NMB stain, RNA and ribosomes that are present in reticulocytes, but not in mature RBCs, stain deeply basophilic (Figure 2.2b). Subtypes of reticulocytes contain different amounts of staining material.
  - Punctate reticulocytes contain only small amounts of blue staining material (Figure 2.2c). Punctate reticulocytes are older reticulocytes and are not typically counted as part of an ongoing regenerative response.
  - Aggregate reticulocytes contain larger clusters of blue staining material (Figure 2.2d). Healthy cats have less than 0.5% aggregate reticulocytes in the peripheral blood. Healthy dogs have less than 1% aggregate reticulocytes in the peripheral blood.
  - Methods for determining the reticulocyte count using NMB can be found at the end of this chapter.
- Mature RBCs of mammals are small, biconcave, eosinophilic cells that lack a nucleus. They contain a large amount of *hemoglobin* (Hb) that contributes to the red coloration of RBCs.
  - There is an area of central pallor in the RBCs of some species, which is caused by the biconcave shape of the erythrocytes.
    - Feline (Figure 2.2e), equine (Figure 2.2g), and bovine (Figure 2.2h) RBCs are relatively small, making it difficult to see central pallor in the RBCs.
    - The diameter of a mature canine RBC is approximately 7.0 mm, which is large enough to appreciate central pallor in canine RBCs (Figure 2.2f).
    - Mature RBCs circulate in blood vessels for approximately 73 days in cats, 100 days in dogs, 145 days in horses, and 160 days in cattle before they are removed from circulation and replaced by newly formed, mature RBCs.
B. Erythrocyte functions
  RBCs are vitally important cells found in all vertebrate animals. RBCs transport O_2 to all cells of the body so that oxidative metabolism can occur. RBCs also transport carbon dioxide (CO_2), a toxic by-product of oxidative metabolism, away from cells. In addition, RBCs help to maintain the pH of the blood within a narrow window to optimize the chemical reactions that occur in the body.
  - The Hb molecules that are present in RBCs allow them to carry O_2 to tissues, help to eliminate CO_2 from the body, and contribute to maintenance of blood pH.

- The amount of Hb in an erythrocyte increases during RBC maturation.
  - Mature RBCs have higher mean cell hemoglobin (MCH) and mean cell hemoglobin concentration (MCHC) parameters than immature RBCs.
- Iron is required for the formation of Hb molecules.
  - Animals with iron deficiency can become anemic because iron is required to produce Hb molecules.
  - Iron is transported in the serum by transferrin molecules. The amount of iron bound to transferrin is the serum iron (SI) concentration.
  - The total iron binding capacity (TIBC) of serum can also be measured. TIBC is a better indicator of the amount of iron available in the body. TIBC indirectly measures the total amount of iron that transferrin will bind. TIBC is increased during iron deficiency in most animals with the exception of dogs.
C. Erythrocyte parameters and indices
  - The number of RBCs present in a blood sample, the size of the RBCs, and the amount of Hb present within the RBCs are examples of erythrocyte parameters and indices that are reported in a CBC.
  - Erythrocyte parameters include hematocrit (Hct), Hb concentration , MCV, MCH, MCHC, and RBC distribution width (RDW).
    - These parameters are used to classify erythrocyte abnormalities and are associated with specific differential diagnoses discussed in more detail in the laboratory data interpretation section of this chapter.
  - PCV is measured after centrifugation of whole blood and indicates the percentage of the blood volume composed of cells (including erythrocytes, leukocytes, and platelets).
    - In practice, PCV is used to estimate Hct. So often, the percentage of blood volume composed of RBCs is determined and the percentage of cells in buffy coat (comprised of leukocytes and platelets) is not included in the measurement.
    - There is a method for determining PCV at the end of this chapter.
  - Hct is the percentage of the blood volume that is composed of erythrocytes. This parameter is calculated by automated analyzers using the formula: Hct (%) = RBC count (millions/μL) × MCV (fL) × 10.
    - The Hct is usually within 1% of the PCV. If the Hct markedly differs from the PCV, the sample should be evaluated for agglutination, leukocytosis, and improper sample handling.
  - Hb is measured by colorimetric techniques or by determining the optical density of oxyhemoglobin in the sample. Automated hematology analyzers report the Hb concentration in a whole blood sample.
    - Hb indicates the oxygen transport capacity of the blood and should be approximately one-third of the Hct.
    - If the Hb:Hct ratio is atypical, a PCV should be performed and reported.
  - The RBC count can be determined using a hemocytometer; however, automated counters are more accurate for mammalian species.
    - Factors that decrease PCV, Hct, Hb, and RBC count include anemia and overhydration.

- Factors that increase PCV, Hct, Hb, and RBC count include dehydration, splenic contraction, and absolute polycythemia.
- Mean corpuscular/cell volume (MCV) is measured directly by automated cell counters. MCV can be calculated using the formula: MCV (fL) = [Hct (%) × 10] ÷ RBC count (millions/μL). The MCV of RBCs varies greatly with species. Patients with a decreased MCV have a microcytosis. The term for an increased MCV is macrocytosis.
  - Microcytosis is often caused by RBC damage or partial lysis. However, several Asian dog breeds naturally have small erythrocytes.
  - Macrocytosis usually indicates that immature erythrocytes are present in the circulation. Greyhound dogs are an exception to this, they naturally have large RBCs. Congenital causes of macrocytosis are also seen. Diseases that affect the bone marrow microenvironment also can increase MCV.
  - Agglutination of RBCs will falsely increase MCV.
- Mean corpuscular/cell hemoglobin concentration (MCHC) is a measurement of RBC hemoglobin content that corrects for RBC volume. It can be calculated using the formula: MCHC (g/dL) = [Hb (g/dL) × 100] ÷ Hct (%). RBCs with a low MCHC are hypochromic. MCHC calculations include intracellular and extracellular Hb. RBCs cannot make excess Hb, so increases in intracellular MCHC are not seen; however, increases in MCHC can be observed when extracellular Hb is increased.
  - Causes of hypochromasia include reticulocytosis, iron deficiency, copper deficiency, and lead toxicity.
  - Causes of hyperchromasia include hemolysis and oxyglobin administration. However true hyperchromasia (a red blood cell containing increased amounts of Hb) does not occur.
- Mean corpuscular hemoglobin (MCH) is the average amount of Hb in RBCs. The calculation for MCH is: MCH (pg) = [Hb (g/dL) × 10] ÷ RBC count (millions/μL). MCH and MCHC are similarly affected by disease.
- Red cell distribution width (RDW) is determined by some automated cell counters. It indicates the degree of anisocytosis (size difference) in RBCs. RDW = [(standard deviation of the MCV) ÷ MCV] × 100. Either microcytosis or macrocytosis may increase RDW.

D. Erythrocyte arrangement
- In healthy animals, RBCs are evenly distributed throughout the monolayer of a blood smear.
- Rouleaux occurs when RBCs are stacked in lines (Figure 2.3a). Rouleaux is commonly seen in blood from healthy cats and disperses when blood is diluted with saline.
  - Increased fibrinogen and globulin concentrations may cause rouleaux.
- Agglutination is the aggregation of RBCs into grape-like clusters (Figure 2.3b). Agglutination is an abnormal finding in any species. Agglutinated RBCs do not disperse when blood is diluted with saline and indicates ongoing immune-mediated disease. The method for performing a saline agglutination test is presented at the end of this chapter.

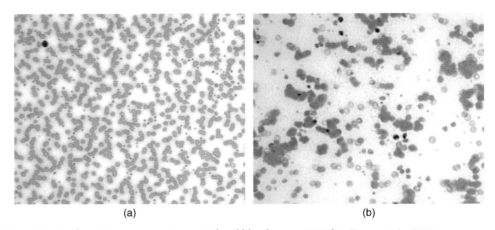

(a)   (b)

Figure 2.3   Erythrocyte arrangements on peripheral blood smears (Wright–Giemsa stain, 200×
magnification). (a) Rouleaux of erythrocytes from a domestic shorthaired cat. (b) Agglutination of
erythrocytes from a Lhasa apso.

E. Erythrocyte morphology
  - Abnormalities in the size and shape of RBCs in a blood smear have been
    associated with specific disease processes. It is critical to report erythrocyte
    morphology on a CBC so that diseases can be accurately diagnosed. The
    following section describes morphological changes that can be observed in
    erythrocytes.
  - Anisocytosis is the term for differences in cell size (Figure 2.4a). In healthy
    patients, RBCs will be the same diameter throughout the blood smear.
    - Anisocytosis may affect specific RBC parameters reported by most automated
      hematology analyzers.
      - RDW is increased.
      - MCV may be abnormal.
        - MCV is decreased if the RBCs are smaller than average.
          - RBCs that are smaller than average may indicate ongoing hemolysis.
        - MCV is increased if the RBCs are larger than average.
          - RBCs that are larger than average are often immature cells called
            reticulocytes.
        - If there is a mixture of both small and large RBCs, the average size of the
          RBCs may be within the reference interval and so MCV will appear
          normal.
  - Polychromasia is the term for cells that stain with both basophilic and
    eosinophilic dyes (Figure 2.4b). RBCs that stain a bluish-red color are immature
    cells called reticulocytes. Compared to mature RBCs, reticulocytes contain a
    large amount of residual RNA and a low amount of Hb. These differences cause
    the blue staining with Romanowski-type stains. Reticulocytes also tend to be
    larger than mature RBCs.
    - Polychromasia is associated with changes in specific RBC parameters.
      - MCH and/or MCHC are typically decreased.

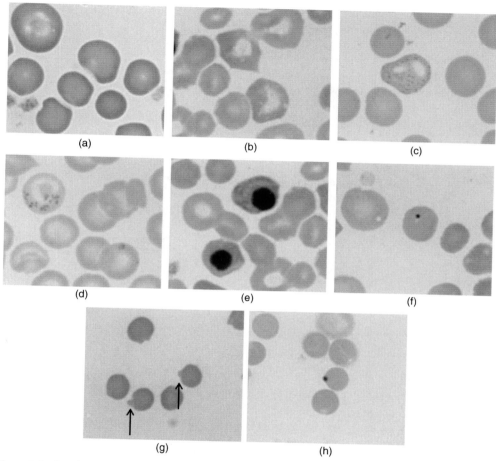

Figure 2.4   Peripheral blood smears illustrating differences in erythrocyte morphology (1400×
magnification). (a–g) Wright–Giemsa stained samples. (a) Anisocytosis (difference in erythrocyte size) in a
Chihuahua. (b) Polychromasia in a Lhasa apso. (c) Basophilic stippling in a Maine coon erythrocyte. (d)
Siderotic plaque (Pappenheimer body) in an erythrocyte from a wire fox terrier. (e) Nucleated red blood cells
(metarubricytes) from a Lhasa apso. (f) Howell--Jolly body in a Lhasa apso erythrocyte. (g) Heinz bodies
(arrows) in domestic shorthaired cat erythrocytes. (h) Erythrocyte containing a Heinz body (blue-staining
defect) in a new methylene blue-stained sample from a domestic shorthaired cat.

- MCV usually is increased.
- Basophilic stippling occurs when dense aggregates of residual RNA remain in
  immature RBCs (Figure 2.4c).
- Siderocytes are RBCs that contain basophilic inclusions consistent with iron
  (Figure 2.4d).
  - It is important to distinguish these inclusions from RBC parasites.
  - Siderocyte inclusions can be confirmed as iron with a special stain such as
    Prussian blue.
- nRBCs are metarubricytes (Figure 2.4e).

- Appropriate nRBC release is observed in strongly regenerative anemia and hypoxic conditions.
- Inappropriate nRBC release is associated with abnormal RBC maturation and diseases of the bone marrow and spleen.
- Howell–Jolly bodies are basophilic nuclear remnants in RBCs (Figure 2.4f).
- Heinz bodies are areas of denatured and precipitated Hb that are caused by oxidative damage to the RBC. Heinz bodies stain pale red with Romanowski-type stains (Figure 2.4g) and stain blue with NMB stain (Figure 2.4h). Heinz body formation can lead to intravascular hemolysis because of the damage to the RBC membrane.
  - Up to 5% Heinz bodies can be present in normal cat blood. Cats are particularly susceptible to Heinz body anemia.
  - Importantly, many animals with Heinz bodies have been exposed to a toxin. Toxins that have been reported to cause Heinz body anemia are listed below.
    - Cats and dogs
      - Acetaminophen (Tylenol®), onion, zinc (pennies, Desitin®), benzocaine, methylene blue, and vitamin K_3
    - Cats
      - Propofol, propylene glycol, phenols, methionine, phenazopyridine, naphthalene (moth balls), and copper
    - Horses
      - Red maple leaf toxicity, phenothiazine
    - Cattle
      - Selenium deficiency, kale
- Poikilocytosis is the term for varied RBC shapes. RBCs of healthy cats, dogs, horses, and cattle appear round on a peripheral blood smear. Specific types of shape changes are associated with specific disease processes. This chapter includes a short list of the most common types of poikilocytosis seen in veterinary medicine. For a more inclusive list, refer to Schalm's Veterinary Hematology.
  - Echinocytes (burr cells and crenated erythrocytes) are the most common type of poikilocyte in a peripheral blood smear. These cells are RBCs that have several evenly spaced spicules (Figure 2.5a). This shape is nearly always due to drying artifact that occurs during preparation of the blood smear.
  - Acanthocytes are RBCs with irregular spicules (Figure 2.5). This type of poikilocyte is caused by an altered ratio of lipid to cholesterol molecules in the RBC membrane.
    - Differential diagnoses include diseases such as liver disease, cancer, and disseminated intravascular coagulation (DIC). DIC is discussed more in Chapter 3.
  - Schistocytes (schizocytes) are RBC fragments that indicate the RBCs have been sheared by intravascular fibrin or turbulent blood flow (Figure 2.5c). They are very important to recognize because of the severity of the diseases that cause their formation.
  - Spherocytes are rounded RBCs with a normal MCV but a smaller appearance on a blood smear (Figure 2.5d). Spherocytes are not evaluated in feline, equine, and bovine blood because the RBC diameter of these species is already

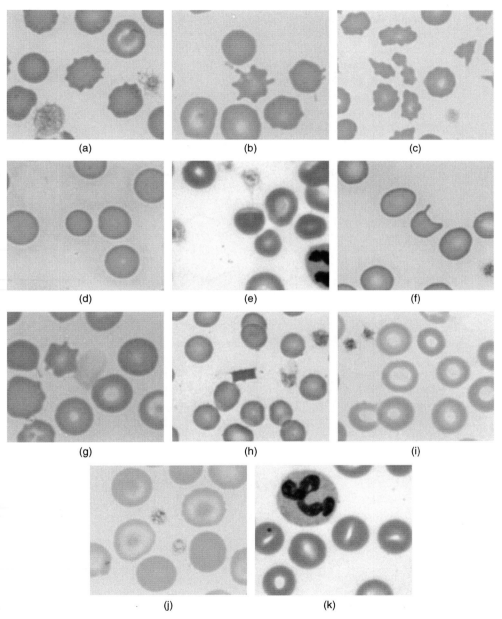

Figure 2.5   Peripheral blood smears depicting erythrocyte poikilocytosis (Wright–Giemsa stain, 1400×
magnification). (a) Ecchinocyte in a great dane. (b) Acanthocyte from a red bone hound. (c) Schistocytes
from a domestic shorthaired cat. (d) Spherocyte from a giant schnauzer. (e) Eccentrocyte from a miniature
pinscher. (f) Keratocyte from a borzoi. (g) Ghost cell caused by intravascular hemolysis in a red bone hound.
(h) Hemoglobin crystal from a domestic longhaired cat. (i) Leptocyte from a shih tzu. (j) Target cells from a
wire fox terrier. (k) Stomatocyte from a miniature pinscher.

small. Spherocytes in dogs are smaller in diameter and lack the central pallor that can be seen in normal canine RBCs. The top differential diagnosis in a dog with large numbers of spherocytosis should be immune-mediated hemolytic anemia (IMHA). However, it is important to remember that other processes have been associated with spherocyte formation including transfusion of stored blood.

- Eccentrocytes are RBCs with Hb condensed to one side of the cell (Figure 2.5e). This is caused by oxidative damage to the Hb molecule. The differentials associated with Heinz body formation are also associated with eccentrocyte formation. Animals with congenital deficiency of enzymes involved in oxidative repair may also have eccentrocytes.
- Keratocytes (helmet cells) contain a torn vesicle to one side of the RBC (Figure 2.5f) and often form during oxidative damage to RBCs.
- Ghost cells are pale remnants of RBCs that are lysed within blood vessels during intravascular hemolysis (Figure 2.5g).
- Hb crystals are angular pieces of Hb that are occasionally seen in blood smears (Figure 2.5h). The clinical significance of these damaged RBCs is not well established.
- Leptocytes are thin RBCs with an increased area of central pallor (Figure 2.5i). These cells often appear folded on themselves.
  - Diseases associated with leptocyte formation include iron deficiency and liver diseases.
- Target cells (codocytes) are leptocytes that look like a target with Hb around the cell edges and at the center of the cell (Figure 2.5j). Differential diagnoses are the same as those that cause leptocyte formation.
- Stomatocytes have a thick ring of Hb around the edges of the RBC and an oval area of central pallor (Figure 2.5k). Differential diagnoses are the same as those that cause leptocyte formation. There is also a hereditary stomatocytosis in dogs.

F. Erythron

The erythron is the portion of a CBC that reports RBC numbers, indices, and/or morphology. Here, the medical terminology used to describe abnormalities in the erythron is discussed.

- Erythrocytosis is an increase in Hct, RBC count, and Hb and may be due to hemoconcentration or polycythemia.
  - Hemoconcentration occurs when the amount of fluid in the blood vessels is decreased.
    - Observed in dehydrated patients.
  - Polycythemia occurs when the numbers of mature erythrocytes produced and released into the peripheral blood are increased.
    - This condition is rare.
- Anemia is defined as a decreased number of RBCs in the peripheral blood. This causes a decrease in Hct, RBC count, and Hb. Many disease processes cause anemia. Overhydration can also decrease Hct, RBC count, and Hb due to the increased amount of fluid in the plasma, which decreases the number of erythrocytes per microliter of blood. Typical clinical signs of anemia include pale

mucous membranes, weakness, tachycardia, syncope, heart murmur, weak pulse, increased sensitivity to cold, and shock. Signalment, patient history, and physical examination are needed to determine the underlying cause of a patient's anemia. Classification of anemia helps narrow down the list of differential diagnoses.

- Classification by bone marrow response separates diseases that cause loss or destruction of erythrocytes from diseases that affect production of erythrocytes.
  - A regenerative response occurs when the bone marrow is responding to the anemia. Erythron findings indicate that immature erythrocytes are being released from the bone marrow and include reticulocytosis, polychromasia, macrocytosis, and hypochromasia.
  - A non-regenerative response is seen when erythropoiesis is not occurring during anemia. Disease processes that prevent normal erythrocyte maturation include iron deficiency, chronic inflammatory disease, renal failure, aplastic anemia, pure red cell aplasia, and endocrinopathies.
- Classification by erythrocyte indices uses specific aspects of RBC morphology (size) and maturity (Hb content) to determine the underlying cause of disease. Classification by RBC size (MCV) and Hb content (MCH and MCHC) is a bit complex and takes WBC and platelet counts into account to determine disease differentials.
  - Although complex, the clinical information provided by MCV, MCH, and MCHC is very important for veterinarians to consider when diagnosing disease in anemic patients.

TECHNICIAN TIP 2–1:

RBC size (MCV)

    RBCs with an MCV within reference limits are normocytic.
    RBCs with a decreased MCV are microcytic.
    RBCs with an increased MCV are macrocytic.

Hb concentration (MCH or MCHC)

    RBCs with an MCH and MCHC within reference limits are normochromic.
    RBCs with a decreased MCH or MCHC are hypochromic.
    RBCs with an increased MCH or MCHC are hyperchromic.

- Note that lipemia and Heinz bodies can artificially increase MCH and MCHC by interfering with the measurement of Hb.
- Classification of anemia by pathophysiology of disease may be difficult to determine from a CBC alone. This classification scheme often requires additional knowledge about the patient. There are three ways that the number of erythrocytes can be decreased in an animal: (1) RBCs can be lost during hemorrhage, (2) RBCs can be destroyed by hemolysis, or (3) RBC production can be decreased.
  - Hemorrhagic anemia is the loss of erythrocytes. Alterations that are detected on a CBC depend on how long the blood loss has been occurring.

- Peracute hemorrhage is a rapid, ongoing loss of blood. Within hours, peracute hemorrhage becomes acute hemorrhage.
  - Patients have a normal Hct due to the concurrent loss of cells and plasma. In addition, splenic contraction releases RBCs into peripheral circulation. Hypovolemic shock occurs if greater than one-third of the animal's blood volume is lost.
- Acute hemorrhage is a recent, rapid loss of blood. Trauma, gastrointestinal (gi) ulceration, and vascular neoplasms are common causes of acute hemorrhage. Thrombocytopenia itself rarely causes acute hemorrhage. However, clotting abnormalities can cause acute hemorrhage.
  - Hct, RBC count, Hb, and plasma protein concentration are decreased a few hours after acute blood loss.
  - Most animals that experience acute hemorrhage mount a strong regenerative response within a few days after the blood loss.

> **TECHNICIAN TIP 2–2:** Remember that a regenerative response is characterized by macrocytic, hypochromic erythrocytes and polychromsia. Reticulocytosis can be confirmed with NMB staining (except in horses).

- If reticulocytosis persists more than 3 weeks, the anemia has become chronic in nature and additional diagnostics are warranted.
- Chronic hemorrhage is associated with a slower onset of anemia. Animals often adjust over time to the decreased oxygen carrying capacity of the blood and do not show overt signs of anemia until the anemia is very severe.
  - Hypoproteinemia and thrombocytosis are commonly seen.
  - The response to chronic anemia is usually mildly regenerative with macrocytosis and hypochromasia. However, iron deficiency anemia with microcytosis and hypochromasia can occur due to continued loss of iron if blood is being lost externally.
  - Occult external blood loss (through the GI tract, urinary tract, or skin) is a common cause of chronic hemorrhage.
- Hemolytic anemia is caused by lysis of RBCs. Diseases that lead to hemolytic anemia often cause rapid destruction of RBCs so clinical signs of anemia can be severe. Hemolysis may occur outside of blood vessels or within vessels but most diseases that cause hemolysis have components of both extravascular and intravascular hemolysis. Hemolysis can increase MCH and/or MCHC.
  - Extravascular hemolysis occurs outside of the peripheral blood. Immune-mediated disease, decreased erythrocyte deformability, reduced erythrocyte metabolism, and/or increased macrophage phagocytic activity can lead to extravascular hemolysis.
    - Findings that may be associated with extravascular hemolysis include reticulocytosis, normal or increased plasma protein concentration, neutrophilia, monocytosis, thrombocytosis, hyperbilirubinemia, splenomegaly, Heinz bodies, RBC parasites, and poikilocytes.

- Intravascular hemolysis occurs within the blood vessels. Causes include complement-mediated lysis of RBCs, physical damage to the RBC membrane, oxidative damage to the RBC membrane, osmotic hemolysis, and hemolysis caused by toxins.
  - Findings that may be associated with intravascular hemolysis include reticulocytosis, hemoglobinemia, icterus, hyperchromasia, increased MCH, hemoglobinuria, hemosiderinuria, hyperbilirubinemia, Heinz bodies, RBC parasites, and poikilocytes.
- Specific diseases or red blood cell pathology resulting in abnormal red blood cell morphology and hemolysis are listed to below.
  - IMHA occurs when antibodies and complement bind antigens on erythrocyte membranes.
    - Both extravascular and intravascular hemolysis can occur.
    - Spherocytosis can be detected in blood samples from some dogs with IMHA.
    - Erythrocyte agglutination may be observed owing to the aggregation of RBCs covered with antibodies.
    - If spherocytes and/or agglutination are not observed in the blood smear from a patient suspected of having IMHA, a Coombs' test can be performed to detect IgG, C_3, or cold-reactive IgM on the RBC membrane (see Methods).
    - Known causes of IMHA include infectious organisms (viral diseases, rickettsial diseases, and RBC parasites), pharmaceuticals, abnormal T-cell function, and paraneoplastic syndromes. In most cases of IMHA in dogs, no underlying cause for the disease is found.
  - Physical damage to RBCs occurs with several disease processes.
    - These diseases induce intravascular hemolysis.
    - Schistocytes (circulating RBC fragments) are commonly observed with this type of damage.
    - Differentials include DIC, vasculitis, hemangiosarcoma, and heartworm disease.
  - Transfusion reactions.
    - Transfusion reactions occur when a patient that has received blood from a donor produces antibodies against the blood group antigens on the donor's RBCs. The antibodies cause lysis of the transfused cells that often leads to death of the patient.
  - Blood groups in cats can cause severe transfusion reactions and neonatal isoerythrolysis.
    - Type A cats are have the A antigen on their RBCs.
      - Anti-B antibodies naturally occur in type A cats but usually only cause increased erythrocyte removal during the first transfusion of B-positive blood.
    - Type B cats have the B antigen on their RBCs.
      - Anti-A antibodies are naturally occurring antibodies in type B cats and cause severe hemolysis when A-positive blood is transfused.

- When type B queens are mated to type A toms, kittens that inherit type A blood from the tom can experience severe hemolysis after nursing.
  - This is termed neonatal isoerythrolysis.
- Type AB cats have both A and B antigens on the RBC surface.
  - These cats do not produce anti-A or anti-B antibodies.
- In dogs, there are approximately 13 blood groups named for different dog erythrocyte antigens (DEAs) on the RBCs. Dogs can be positive for more than one blood group (for example, a dog could be DEA-1.1, DEA-3, and DEA-7 positive).
  - DEA-1.1 and 1.2 are of primary importance. During transfusion with mismatched blood, patients can form antibodies against these DEA antigens. If a second transfusion of mismatched blood is given, severe hemolysis will occur.
  - Dogs that are DEA-4 positive only are considered universal donors.
- Horses have over 34 blood factors that are placed into 7 blood groups (A, C, D, K, P, Q, and U). Typically, the first mismatched blood transfusion will cause hemolysis but not a severe transfusion reaction in horses. However, blood types Aa & Qa are important because antibodies against these antigens are naturally occurring and can cause neonatal isoerythrolysis.
  - Neonatal isoerythrolysis occurs in Aa or Qa negative mares with their second Aa or Qa positive foal. Ingestion of colostrum containing anti-Aa or anti-Qa antibodies causes severe hemolysis in the foal.
- Cattle have over 80 blood factors that are placed into 11 blood groups (A, B, C, F, J, L, M, S, Z, R', and T'). Similar to horses, the first mismatched blood transfusion will cause mild hemolysis.
- To prevent unwanted transfusion reactions, blood should be properly crossmatched. (See the crossmatch method at the end of this chapter.).
  - The major crossmatch combines the patient's serum with the donor's RBCs to detect antibodies in the patient that will lyse the donor's RBCs. This is very important to avoid lysis of the transfused blood cells.
  - The minor crossmatch combines the patient's RBCs with the donor's serum to determine if the donor has antibodies that will lyse the patient's RBCs. This is of less importance because the donor's antibodies will be diluted out by the patient's blood once the transfusion is given.
  - Incompatible crossmatches cause hemolysis and/or agglutination of the sample.

Leukocytes

A. Leukocyte maturation
   White blood cells are important components of the immune system. The subtypes of leukocytes typically observed in the peripheral blood include *neutrophils*, *eosinophils*, *basophils*, *monocytes*, and *lymphocytes*.
   - An abnormal leukocyte count in the peripheral blood is a key indication of disease in animals.

- Neutrophils, eosinophils, and basophils are subtypes of granulocytes, which are derived from myeloid cells that originate in hematopoietic organs from a common precursor cell called a myeloblast.
- Granulocytes mature in the bone marrow and other hematopoietic organs until they are released into the peripheral blood. It takes two to seven days to produce a mature granulocyte. The process of granulocyte maturation is called myelopoiesis.
- As granulocytes mature, the cells become smaller, cytoplasmic granules begin to pick up Romanowski-type stains, and the nucleus condenses and eventually appears segmented.
  - Myeloblasts are the first microscopically identifiable myeloid precursor. They are large cells that, when stained with Romanowski-type stains, have basophilic cytoplasm and a rounded nucleus with a prominent nucleolus (Figure 2.6a).
    - These cells mature into promyelocytes that may eventually form neutrophils, eosinophils, or basophils.
  - Promyelocytes are similar in size to myeloblasts and contain small pink granules within a lightly basophilic cytoplasm. The nucleus of a promyelocyte

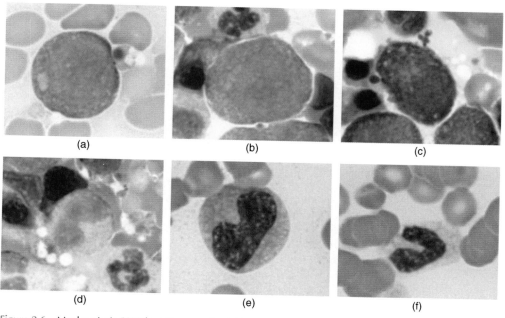

(a)   (b)   (c)

(d)   (e)   (f)

Figure 2.6   Myelopoiesis (Wright–Giemsa stain, 1400× magnification). (a–d) Bone marrow aspirate from a Bernese mountain dog. (a) Myeloblast with basophilic cytoplasm and a large, rounded nucleus containing several nucleoli. (b) Promyelocyte with basophilic cytoplasm; small, eosinophilic, cytoplasmic granules; and a round nucleus. (c) Eosinophil myelocyte with relatively abundant basophilic cytoplasm; numerous, large, brightly eosinophilic granules; and a round, eccentrically located nucleus. (d) Neutrophil metamyelocyte with pale cytoplasm and a thick, cleaved nucleus. (e and f) Peripheral blood smear from a cocker spaniel. (e) Neutrophil metamyelocyte with cytoplasmic basophilia and a thick, cleaved nucleus. (f) Band neutrophil with pale cytoplasm and a horseshoe-shaped nucleus.

is rounded and may contain a nucleolus (Figure 2.6b). These cells mature into myelocytes.

- Myelocytes are smaller than promyelocytes and have lightly basophilic cytoplasm and a rounded nucleus that is smaller than the nucleus of a promyelocyte. At this stage, the cells can be specifically subdivided to reflect the type of granulocyte they will become.
  - Neutrophil myelocytes do not contain visible cytoplasmic granules.
  - Eosinophil myelocytes contain pink/red/orange (eosinophilic) cytoplasmic granules (Figure 2.6c).
  - Basophil myelocytes contain blue/purple (basophilic) cytoplasmic granules.
- Metamyelocytes are smaller than myelocytes and have lightly basophilic cytoplasm and a cleaved nucleus. These cells are subdivided into neutrophil, eosinophil, or basophil metamyelocytes based on the type of cytoplasmic granules they contain.
  - A neutrophil metamyelocyte from a bone marrow aspirate is shown in Figure 2.6d.
  - Metamyelocytes are rarely released into the peripheral blood (Figure 2.6e). Neutrophil metamyelocytes in the peripheral blood may indicate that an animal has a severe inflammatory disease.
- Band neutrophils, band eosinophils, and band basophils are slightly smaller than metamyelocytes. They have lightly basophilic cytoplasm and a horseshoe-shaped nucleus. In addition, band eosinophils contain eosinophilic granules and band basophils contain basophilic granules.
  - A band neutrophil from a peripheral blood smear is shown in Figure 2.6f.
  - Release of increased numbers of band neutrophils into the peripheral blood is called a left shift and often is associated with severe inflammatory disease.
- Mature granulocytes have clear to lightly basophilic cytoplasm and a segmented nucleus with a dense chromatin pattern.
  - Segmented neutrophils are the predominant leukocyte in the peripheral blood of feline, canine, and equine patients.
    - Neutrophils contain granules that are neutral-staining with Romanowski-type stains, therefore their granules are not seen microscopically (Figure 2.7 a–d).
    - Neutrophils circulate in the peripheral blood for 7–14 hours and can live in tissues for 24–48 hours.
    - Neutrophils are extremely important for the elimination of bacterial organisms from infected tissues.
  - Eosinophils are present in low numbers and sometimes completely absent in the peripheral blood of healthy animals.
    - Eosinophils contain granules that stain pink to red with Romanowski-type stains. The shape of the granules varies slightly in different species.
      - Feline eosinophils have numerous, small, rice-shaped, pink to orange granules (Figure 2.7e).
      - Canine and bovine eosinophils have numerous, small, round, pink granules (Figure 2.7f and h, respectively).

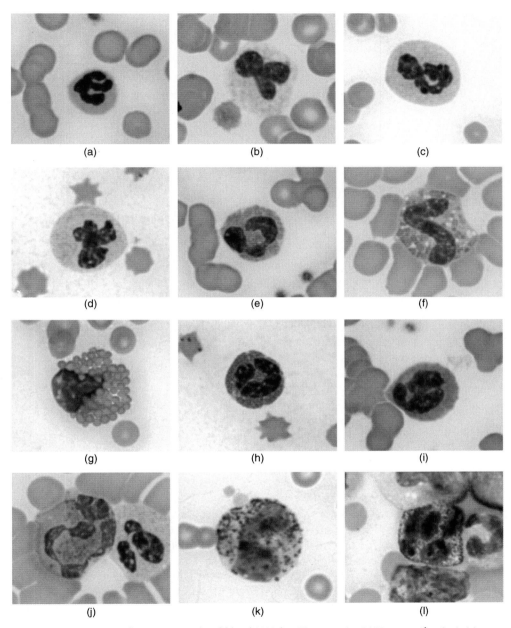

Figure 2.7   Mature granulocytes in peripheral blood (Wright–Giemsa stain, 1400× magnification). (a) Feline-segmented neutrophil. (b) Segmented neutrophil from a cocker spaniel. (c) Segmented neutrophil from a foal. (d) Bovine segmented neutrophil. (e) Eosinophil from a domestic shorthaired cat. (f) Canine eosinophil. (g) Eosinophil from a foal. (h) Bovine eosinophil. (i) Basophil from a domestic shorthaired cat. (j) Basophil from a mixed-breed dog. (k) Basophil from a foal. (L) Basophil from a Jersey cow.

- Equine eosinophils have many large, round, pink granules (Figure 2.7g).
- Eosinophils have a short half-life of approximately 30 minutes in circulation.
- Eosinophil numbers will often increase in circulation in response to parasitic organisms.
  - Basophils are rarely seen in the peripheral blood of healthy animals.
    - In most species, basophils contain granules that stain blue to purple with Romanowski-type stains.
      - Feline basophil granules are numerous, large, round, and stain lavender (Figure 2.7i).
      - Canine basophil granules appear scarce, small, angular, and stain purple. The cytoplasm of canine basophils may stain more purple than blue (Figure 2.7j).
      - Equine and bovine basophils contain many small, round, purple, cytoplasmic granules (Figure 2.7k and l, respectively).
    - The half-life of a basophil in circulation is 6 hours. They survive longer in tissues.
    - Basophils are associated with allergic disease and parasitism.
- Monocytes are histiocytic cells of the mononuclear phagocyte system that circulate in the peripheral blood. Monocytes originate from precursor cells in the bone marrow and other hematopoietic organs. However, monocyte precursors are present in very low numbers and cannot be identified using morphological characteristics alone. As monocytes leave the blood stream and enter the tissues, they differentiate into several types of histiocytes, including macrophages and dendritic cells.
  - Monocytes appear slightly larger than segmented neutrophils and have blue-gray cytoplasm and a round, cleaved, or irregularly shaped nucleus (Figure 2.8 a–d). Monocytes often contain low numbers of clear cytoplasmic vacuoles.
  - Monocytes are present in low numbers in the peripheral blood of healthy mammals and circulate for approximately 24 hours. They survive in tissues for an extended period of time.
  - Monocytes often are associated with chronic inflammatory disease.
- Lymphocytes are found in moderate numbers in the peripheral blood of cats, dogs, and horses and in significant numbers in bovine peripheral blood. Lymphocytes reside in lymph nodes, spleen, thymus, tonsils, bone marrow, and other lymphoid tissues throughout the body. They are long-lived and can circulate into and out of the peripheral blood.
  - Typical circulating small lymphocytes are smaller than neutrophils and have scant lightly basophilic cytoplasm and a round nucleus with a dense chromatin pattern (Figure 2.9 a–d).
  - Lymphocytes can be subdivided into B-lymphocytes and T-lymphocytes using immunologic techniques such as immunocytochemistry and flow cytometry.
    - T-lymphocytes (T-cells) stimulate the immune response to infection and eliminate cells that contain intracellular pathogens.

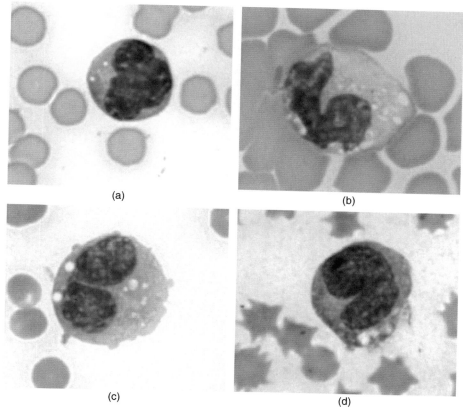

Figure 2.8   Monocytes in peripheral blood (Wright–Giemsa stain, 1400x magnification). (a) Monocyte from a domestic shorthaired cat. (b) Canine monocyte. (c) Monocyte from a foal. (d) Bovine monocyte.

- T-cell maturation occurs in the thymus.
- T-cells replicate in lymphoid organs when stimulated by a pathogen.
- B-lymphocytes (B-cells) produce antibodies to help fight infection.
  - B-cell maturation was first discovered in birds and occurs in the bursa of Fabricius.
  - In mammals, B-cells mature in the bone marrow and lymphoid tissues.
  - B-cells replicate in lymphoid organs when an animal is exposed to a pathogen.

B. Leukocyte functions

As mentioned previously, leukocytes are important cells of the immune system. Leukocytes leave the peripheral blood vessels and migrate into tissues in response to chemotactic signals at sites of inflammation.

- The primary neutrophil chemoattractant released during an inflammatory response is interleukin-8 (IL-8). Once in the tissue, neutrophil functions include the following:
  - Phagocytosis of microorganisms

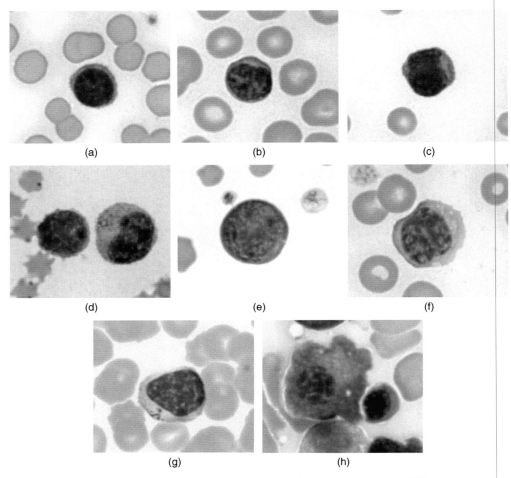

Figure 2.9   Lymphocytes (Wright–Giemsa stain, 1400× magnification). (a–g) Peripheral blood smears. (a) Small lymphocyte from a domestic shorthaired cat. (b) Small lymphocyte from a mixed-breed dog. (c) Small lymphocyte from a foal. (d) Small lymphocyte (left) and large granular lymphocyte (right) from a Jersey cow. (e) Feline reactive lymphocyte. (f) Atypical lymphocyte from a mixed-breed dog. (g) Large granular lymphocyte from a golden retriever. (h) Plasma cell in a bone marrow aspirate from a Bernese mountain dog.

- Secretion of anti-microbial enzymes and pro-inflammatory molecules (cytokines)
- Production of an oxidative burst that generates free radicals that are anti-microbial
- Eosinophils migrate toward high concentrations of IL-5 in injured tissues. Eosinophil functions include the following:
  - Defense against helminthic parasites
  - Secretion of molecules that modulate the inflammatory response
  - Contribution to asthma and allergic diseases
  - Limited phagocytosis of microorganisms

- Basophils also migrate toward IL-5, but there are very low numbers of these cells in the body. Their functions are similar to mast cell functions and include the following:
  - Histamine release during allergic hypersensitivity reactions
  - Limited anti-parasitic activity
- Monocytes become macrophages as they migrate into tissues. These cells are critical for the induction of fully functional immune responses. Macrophage functions include the following:
  - Antigen presentation
    - Antigen (Ag) segments are bound to major histocompatibility complex (MHC) proteins.
    - MHC:Ag complexes are moved to the surface of the macrophage and are presented to T-cells.
  - Production of cytokines that regulate the immune response
  - Phagocytosis of dead cells and microorganisms
- Lymphocytes are subdivided into several cell types based on their function.
  - T-cells produce cytokines that regulate the immune response. Several important aspects of the immune response are dependent on T-cell function including the following:
    - Activation and differentiation of B-cells
    - T-cell proliferation
    - Lysis of cells infected with virus
    - Suppression of inappropriate immune responses
  - B-cells produce antibodies that help eliminate and protect against pathogens.

C. Leukocyte parameters

The total number of leukocytes, WBC differential cell counts, and morphology of leukocytes are examples of leukocyte parameters.

- WBC count per microliter of blood
  - Animals with low WBC counts are leukopenic.
  - Animals with high WBC counts have a leukocytosis.
- The WBC differential determines the percentage of different leukocyte subsets present in the sample.
  - Cell percentage is converted into an absolute differential count by multiplying the percentage of each cell type by the total number of leukocytes in the sample. An example of this calculation is given in Table 2.2.
  - Variations in the absolute number of neutrophils, monocytes, lymphocytes, eosinophils, or basophils in a microliter of peripheral blood are associated with various disease processes that are discussed later in the laboratory data interpretation section of this chapter.

D. Leukocyte morphology

Changes in the appearance of the leukocytes are important to report on a CBC.

- Alterations in the nuclear and cytoplasmic characteristics of granulocytes can indicate disease. Most morphological changes are observed in neutrophils.
  - Nuclear changes tend to reflect the maturation of the granulocytes.

Table 2.2　Calculation of absolute leukocyte counts when the total white blood cell (WBC) count is 15,000 cells/μL.

	Percentage of Each Cell in a 200-Cell Differential Count	Formula to Calculate Absolute Cell Counts	Calculated Absolute Cell Counts
	(No. of Cells ÷200) × 100 = % of cells	(No. of Cells ÷100) × total WBC count =	(Cells/uL)
Neutrophil	(150/200) × 100 = 75%	75%/100 × 15,000 =	11,250
Lymphocyte	(32/200) × 100 = 16%	16%/100 × 15,000 =	2,400
Monocyte	(16/200) × 100 = 8%	8%/100 × 15,000 =	1,200
Eosinophil	(2/200) × 100 = 1%	1%/100 × 15,000 =	150
Basophil	(0/200) × 100 = 0%	0%/100 × 15,000 =	0

- In healthy mammals, neutrophil, eosinophil, and basophil nuclei have condensed chromatin and contain a few indentations that cause segmentation of the nucleus.
- Granulocytes are hypersegmented when there are more than five nuclear segments (Figure 2.10a). This occurs in neutrophils that have been in circulation too long but is rare to see in eosinophils or basophils.
  - Neutrophil hypersegmentation has been reported in animals with an increased serum cortisol concentration.
- Immature granulocytes are hyposegmented. The nuclear chromatin of immature granulocytes is less condensed than mature cells. Early release of neutrophils from the bone marrow raises concern for a severe inflammatory disease process. An increased number of band neutrophils is called a left shift.
- Pelger–Huet anomaly is a rare congenital condition in which all granulocytes have a hyposegmented nucleus with dense, mature-looking chromatin (Figure 2.10b and c). Cells from animals with Pelger–Huet anomaly function normally and should not be reported as bands.
- Abnormal staining characteristics of the cytoplasm of neutrophils indicate disease. The most common abnormalities occur in patients with severe inflammatory diseases resulting from accelerated production by the bone marrow called toxic changes. Most other abnormalities are inherited diseases and are rarely seen.
  - Toxic changes occur with severe inflammatory diseases.
    - Döhle bodies are small blue-gray cytoplasmic inclusions (Figure 2.10d). Low numbers of these inclusions are common to observe in neutrophils of healthy cats.
    - Cytoplasmic basophilia is a more severe toxic change that is not seen in healthy cats, dogs, horses, or cattle. Döhle bodies and basophilic cytoplasm can be observed within the same cell (Figure 2.10e).

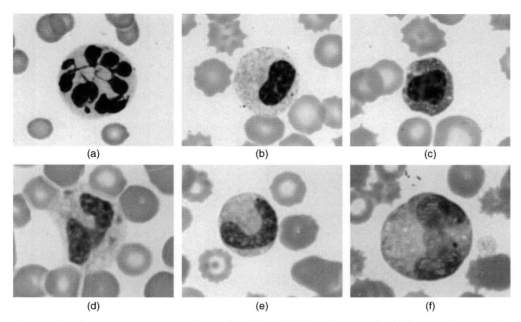

(a)   (b)   (c)

(d)   (e)   (f)

Figure 2.10   Granulocyte morphology in peripheral blood (Wright–Giemsa stain, 1400× magnification). (a) Hypersegmented neutrophil from a domestic longhaired cat. (b and c) Pelger–Huet anomaly in an Australian shepherd. (b) Hyposegmented neutrophil with mature chromatin. (c) Hyposegmented mature eosinophil. (d) Segmented neutrophil with three Döhle bodies from a cocker spaniel. (e) Band neutrophil with cytoplasmic basophilia from a domestic shorthaired cat. (f) Giant neutrophil from a domestic shorthaired cat with cytoplasmic basophilia and vacuolation consistent with a 3–4+ toxic change.

- Cytoplasmic vacuolation in granulocytes is an even more severe indication of toxicity. If this is a true finding (not an artifact of sample preparation), neutrophils will contain Döhle bodies and have basophilic cytoplasm as well as cytoplasmic vacuolation (Figure 2.10f).
- Toxic granulation may occur if primary granules in a neutrophil accumulate eosinophilic stain.
- Inherited diseases with abnormal staining of granulocyte cytoplasm.
  - Patients with Chediak-Higashi syndrome have hypopigmented skin, hair, and eyes. Their granulocytes contain large cytoplasmic granules. Clinical signs of disease are associated with thrombocytopathy (see Chapter 3).
  - Lysosomal storage disorders are caused by alterations in cellular metabolism that prevent normal processing and/or storage of intracellular proteins.
    - Large cytoplasmic granules can be seen in white blood cells of patients with mucopolysaccharide storage diseases.
    - Abnormal vacuolation may be observed in multiple cell types of patients with other types of storage diseases.
    - Lysosomal storage diseases commonly cause mental deterioration.
- Monocyte morphology. Few alterations in monocyte morphology occur with disease.

- Cytoplasmic vacuolation may be increased in animals with inflammatory diseases including ehrlichiosis or erythrocyte parasitism.
- Lymphocyte morphology. Significant morphological differences occur in lymphocytes during disease.
  - Reactive lymphocytes are larger than small lymphocytes and have deeply basophilic cytoplasm. The nuclear chromatin is often clumped (Figure 2.9e). They can be difficult to distinguish from neoplastic lymphoid cells.
    - These cells commonly are observed following antigenic stimulation.
  - Atypical lymphocytes have more abundant cytoplasm than small lymphocytes. The cytoplasm is lightly basophilic and the nucleus is round or cleaved, small, and dense (Figure 2.9f).
    - These cells often are an insignificant finding. Low numbers of atypical lymphocytes can be associated with antigenic stimulation but high numbers of atypical lymphocytes may be associated with chronic lymphoid leukemia.
  - Large granular lymphocytes (LGLs) are cytotoxic T-cells or natural killer (NK) cells that can be observed in small numbers in the peripheral blood. These cells are slightly larger and have more abundant cytoplasm than a small lymphocyte. Small eccentrically located metachromatic (purple- or fuchsia-staining) granules are present in the cytoplasm of these cells (Figure 2.9d and g).
    - LGLs may indicate that there is ongoing antigenic stimulation by an intracellular organism (such as a virus).
    - If LGLs are the predominant type of lymphocyte in the sample and lymphocyte numbers are increased, a neoplastic proliferation of lymphocytes should be considered.
  - Plasma cells are highly differentiated B-cells that are rarely observed in the peripheral blood. They produce a large amount of antibody. Plasma cells have a small eccentrically placed nucleus and abundant deeply basophilic cytoplasm with a prominent clear zone to one side of the nucleus (Figure 2.9h).
    - Marked antigenic stimulation may cause these cells to circulate in the peripheral blood.

E. Leukon

The leukon is the section of a CBC that describes abnormalities in WBC counts and differentials that are indicative of the type of immune response occurring in the patient. Consequently, the type of disease process inducing the immune response can be deduced if the WBC differential is known. Classification of different WBC abnormalities allows for proper assessment and communication of underlying disease differentials in the patient.

- Neutrophilia
  - Increased numbers of circulating neutrophils compared to reference intervals.
  - Neutrophilia may indicate stress, physiological response, or inflammation.
    - Stress leukon
      - Mature neutrophilia, lymphopenia, and eosinopenia
      - Monocytosis also may occur in dogs.
      - Glucocorticoid mediated (exogenous or endogenous). Chronically ill patients will likely develop a stress leukon.

- Physiological leukocytosis
  - Mild neutrophilia and lymphocytosis
  - Animals also may have an increased PCV, hyperglycemia, and increased numbers of RBCs with Howell–Jolly bodies.
  - Induced by epinephrine release due to fear or excitement
  - This change is most common in young cats.
- Inflammatory leukon
  - Most patients have a neutrophilia with or without a left shift.
  - Left shifting occurs if tissue demand is high.
    - If tissue demand far exceeds the ability of the bone marrow to produce neutrophils, neutrophil counts can fall below reference intervals.
  - Toxic changes, lymphopenia, and/or eosinopenia may or may not be observed.
  - There is often a monocytosis and an increased fibrinogen concentration.
    - In horses and cattle, elevated fibrinogen is a much more sensitive indicator of inflammation than changes in the leukon.
  - Caused by infectious or non-infectious inflammatory disorders
- Neutrophilia due to chronic myeloid leukemia is rare.
- Neutropenia
  - Decrease in the number of neutrophils compared to a species-specific reference interval.
  - Caused by severe inflammation or bone marrow damage.
    - Peracute inflammation will cause neutropenia if neutrophils are used before granulopoiesis can occur.
    - Overwhelming infection (such as bacterial mastitis, salmonellosis, peritonitis, and pyometra) can require more neutrophils than the body can supply.
    - Panleukopenia in cats and parvovirus in dogs cause destruction of cells in the bone marrow and increased tissue demand in the gut.
    - Drug reactions may cause neutropenia due to bone marrow damage. Bone marrow cytology and histopathology may be beneficial in these patients.
    - Cyclic hematopoiesis (Gray Collie Syndrome) is caused by an autosomal recessive genetic defect in collie dogs with gray hair coats.
      - Animals have cyclic fluctuations in the numbers of WBCs and platelets.
      - Neutrophil counts drop dangerously low every 10–11 days.
        - This leaves the animal prone to bacterial infection.
    - If all other causes of neutropenia are ruled out, immune-mediated destruction of neutrophils should be considered.
- Eosinophilia
  - Increase in the number of eosinophils compared to a species-specific reference interval.
  - Etiologies include GI parasites, heartworm, lungworm, flea infestation, allergic or hypersensitivity reactions, paraneoplastic responses, eosinophilic leukemia, and hypereosinophilic syndrome.

- Eosinopenia
  - Decreased numbers of eosinophils compared to a species-specific reference interval
  - Not usually a relevant finding
  - Stress is a likely cause if there is concurrent neutrophilia and lymphopenia.
- Basophilia
  - Increase in the number of basophils compared to a species-specific reference interval.
  - Differential diagnoses include allergic responses, heartworm disease, GI parasites, hyperlipidemic states, and paraneoplastic responses.
- A decreased number of basophils is not clinically relevant.
- Monocytosis
  - Reported when there are increased numbers of monocytes compared to reference intervals.
  - Often observed with neutrophilia and associated with chronic inflammatory diseases.
- A decreased number of monocytes is not clinically relevant.
- Lymphocytosis
  - The lymphocyte count is increased above the reference interval for that species.
  - Any chronic antigenic stimulation can cause a lymphocytosis particularly *Ehrlichia canis* infection, vaccination, and protozoal infections.
  - Chronic lymphoid leukemia can cause a lymphocytosis. There may or may not be increased numbers of atypical lymphocytes in these patients. Additional diagnostic tests are needed to confirm the diagnosis of chronic lymphoid leukemia.
  - Acute lymphoid leukemia and stage V lymphoma should be suspected in patients with a marked lymphocytosis when large numbers of lymphoblasts are present. Lymphoblasts are large lymphocytes with an immature nucleus; the nuclear diameter is greater than the diameter of a neutrophil and prominent nucleoli can be observed (Figure 2.14b).
- Lymphopenia
  - Decreased numbers of lymphocytes compared to a species-specific reference interval
  - Increased corticosteroid levels commonly cause lymphopenia. Immunosuppression and loss of lymphocyte-rich fluid are less common causes of lymphopenia.

Platelets

A. Platelet maturation

Platelets (thrombocytes) function in hemostasis. Platelets are needed to prevent blood loss during illness or injury. They are a very important component of the peripheral blood and always need to be assessed when reporting data for a CBC.

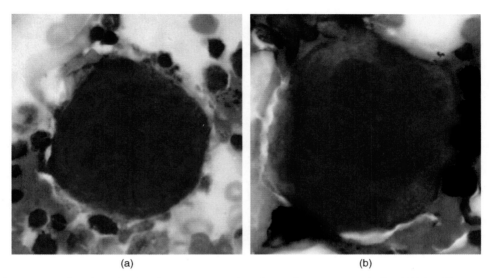

(a)   (b)

Figure 2.11   Thrombopoiesis in a bone marrow aspirate from a Bernese mountain dog (Wright–Giemsa stain, 1000× magnification). (a) Immature megakaryocyte with scant basophilic cytoplasm and a single, large, round nucleus. (b) Mature megakaryocyte with lightly basophilic cytoplasm and a large, multilobulated nucleus.

- Platelets originate in the bone marrow and other hematopoietic organs. The process of platelet maturation is called thrombopoiesis. Platelet production is driven by thrombopoietin.
  - Platelet precursors are called megakaryocytes. Very immature megakaryocytes are large cells with abundant lightly basophilic cytoplasm and a round nucleus with a stippled chromatin pattern (Figure 2.11a). As these cells develop, they become larger and their nucleus becomes multilobulated (Figure 2.11a).
  - Platelets in the circulation of mammals are small 2–4 μm fragments of cytoplasm released from megakaryocytes (Figure 2.12 a-d).
    - The lifespan of a circulating platelet is approximately 5–10 days.
    - The spleen contains a storage pool of platelets that can be released into the peripheral blood during splenic contraction.
    - Mean platelet volume (MPV) may be increased during a regenerative bone marrow response due to early release of large platelets.
B. Platelet functions
  - Hemostasis is the primary function of platelets and is discussed in Chapter 3.
  - Platelets also secrete chemotactic factors and play a key role in initiating inflammation.
C. Platelet parameters
    The major platelet parameters are the platelet count and the MPV. A discussion of the diseases associated with abnormalities in these parameters can be found in Chapter 3.
  - Platelet count per microliter of blood
    - Animals with low platelet counts are thrombocytopenic.
    - Animals with high platelet counts have a thrombocytosis.

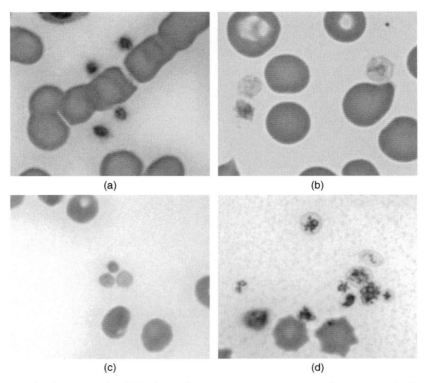

(a)   (b)

(c)   (d)

Figure 2.12   Platelets in peripheral blood (Wright–Giemsa stain, 2114× magnification). (a) Platelets from a domestic shorthaired cat. (b) Platelets from a Chihuahua. (c) Platelets from a foal. (d) Platelets from a Jersey cow.

- The MPV is determined by automated hematology analyzers. MPV is an indication of the size of the platelets in the sample and may be artificially increased if platelet clumps are present.
D. Platelet morphology
  - Microplatelets are even smaller than normal platelets and may be observed with iron-deficiency anemia, immune-mediated disease, or bone marrow aplasia.
  - Large platelets or giant platelets are approximately the diameter of an erythrocyte and are indicative of a regenerative response by megakaryocytes in hematopoietic organs (Figure 2.13a).
  - Megalocytic platelets are larger than the diameter of several erythrocytes and are an indication of bone marrow disease (Figure 2.13b).
E. Thrombon
  The thrombon is the portion of a CBC that describes platelet count, parameters, and morphology. Disease processes associated with platelet counts and MPV outside of the reference intervals are discussed in more detail in Chapter 3.
  - Thrombocytosis is the term for increased numbers of circulating platelets.
    - Patients with markedly increased platelet counts may be at risk for thromboembolism.

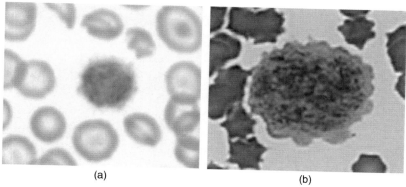

(a)   (b)

Figure 2.13   Atypical platelet morphology in peripheral blood smears (Wright–Giemsa stain, 1960×
magnification). (a) Giant platelet in a peripheral blood smear from a rottweiler. (b) Megalocytic platelet.

- Causes of thrombocytosis include splenic contraction, inflammation, and
  hemorrhage.
  - During hemorrhage, platelets are utilized and lost which triggers a
    regenerative response from the bone marrow to increase platelet numbers.
    - MPV may be increased during a regenerative bone marrow response due
      to early release of large platelets.
  - The presence of increased numbers of abnormal platelets in the peripheral
    blood may indicate bone marrow disease.
- Thrombocytopenia is the term for decreased numbers of circulating platelets.
  - Thrombocytopenia occurs when platelets are destroyed or damaged, lost or
    used too rapidly, or not produced quickly enough.
  - Specific diseases associated with thrombocytopenia are discussed in Chapter 3.

Atypical Cells in the Peripheral Blood

A. Mast cells are round cells that have pale cytoplasm and contain multiple small
   metachromatic (purple-staining) cytoplasmic granules. They have a round,
   centrally located nucleus (Figure 2.14a). These cells usually reside in tissues. The
   presence of mast cells in the peripheral blood is termed mastocythemia.
   - Mastocythemia may be seen in animals with inflammation, allergic disease, or
     mast cell tumors.
B. Blasts are circulating neoplastic cells that are observed in animals with leukemia or
   other cancers that have metastasized to the bone marrow. These diseases disrupt
   the bone marrow microenvironment, so there often is concurrent non-regenerative
   anemia, neutropenia, and/or thrombocytopenia.
   - Acute lymphoid leukemia typically causes a marked increase in lymphocyte
     numbers (lymphocytosis) composed of immature circulating lymphocytes.
     Immature lymphocytes (lymphoblasts) are larger than mature lymphocytes and

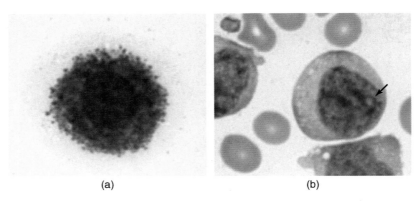

(a)   (b)

Figure 2.14   Abnormal cells in peripheral blood (Wright–Giemsa stain, 1400× magnification). (a) Feline mast cell with rounded cytoplasm (filled with small, metachromatic granules) and a round nucleus. (b) Blast with a moderate amount of basophilic cytoplasm and a rounded nucleus with a prominent nucleolus (arrow) from a mixed-breed dog.

have a moderate amount of basophilic cytoplasm and a round or irregular nucleus with a prominent nucleolus (Figure 2.14b).
- Stage V lymphoma originates from neoplastic lymphocytes in the peripheral lymphoid organs. Neoplastic lymphocytes metastasize to the bone marrow and circulate in the peripheral blood. The peripheral blood of patients with stage V lymphoma can appear nearly identical to that of patients with acute lymphoid leukemia.
  - These patients often have enlarged peripheral lymph nodes, splenomegaly, hepatomegaly, or a mediastinal mass.
- Acute myeloid leukemia is associated with the release of large numbers of myeloblasts from the bone marrow into the peripheral blood.
- Acute monocytic leukemias are rare. With this disease, immature histiocytic cells are observed in high numbers in the peripheral blood. These cells have abundant basophilic cytoplasm and a round nucleus with a prominent nucleolus. They cannot be distinguished from myeloblasts without specialized diagnostic tests.
- Acute megakaryocytic leukemia is a rare neoplasm of platelet precursors that can cause abnormal platelets to be seen in the peripheral blood.

Blood Parasites

Organisms that infect blood cells appear as inclusions in the cytoplasm of the cells on a peripheral blood smear when stained with Romanowski-type stains. Other blood parasites can be found free in the circulation. This section provides the reader with images of the most commonly seen parasites in the United States. Please refer to a veterinary parasitology textbook for more information about the life cycles of these organisms.

A. Blood parasites of cats
- Intracellular RBC pathogens in cats tend to be small piriform structures with a small amount of clear, rounded cytoplasm and an eccentrically located, pinpoint, round, basophilic nucleus.

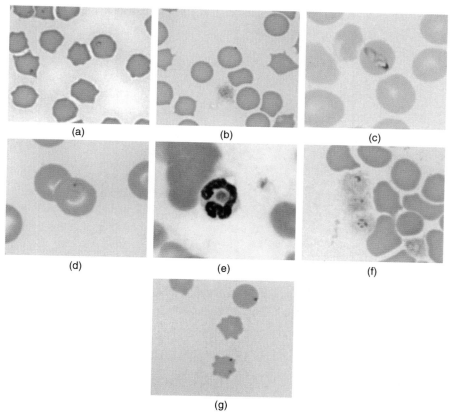

(a)   (b)   (c)

(d)   (e)   (f)

(g)

Figure 2.15   Peripheral blood parasites (Wright-Giemsa stain). (a–f) 1400× magnification. (a) *Cytauxzoon felis* – intracellular piriform-shaped organisms in erythrocytes of a domestic shorthaired cat. (b) *Mycoplasma haemofelis* – extracellular pinpoint organism on an erythrocyte of a domestic shorthaired cat. (c) *Babesia canis* – large intracellular piriform-shaped pathogen in an erythrocyte from a dog. (d) *Babesia gibsoni* – intracellular piriform-shaped pathogen in an erythrocyte from a pit bull terrier. (e) *Ehrlichia ewingii* – round, granular, intracellular organism in the cytoplasm of a neutrophil from a rottweiler. (f) *Anaplasma platys* – small, round to irregular organisms staining deeply basophilic within platelets from a mixed-breed dog. (g) *Anaplasma marginale* – small, round, extracellular pathogens on the erythrocytes of a Jersey cow.

- The organisms listed in the following are transmitted by ticks and bite wounds.
  - *Cytauxzoon felis* (Figure 2.15a)
  - *Babesia cati*
  - *Babesia felis*
- Epicellular RBC pathogens in cats are tiny, basophilic cocci or rings located on the edge of the erythrocyte.
- *Mycoplasma* spp. may be transmitted by fleas and other biting insects.
  - *Mycoplasma haemofelis* (Figure 2.15b)
  - *Mycoplasma haemominutium*
B. Blood parasites of dogs
  - Intracellular pathogens

- *Babesia canis* is transmitted by ticks. It infects RBCs and is a relatively large piriform to tear-drop-shaped structure with clear cytoplasm and an eccentrically located, round, basophlic nucleus (Figure 2.15c).
- *Babesia gibsoni* is transmitted by ticks. It infects RBCs and appears as a small piriform structure with a small amount of clear, rounded cytoplasm and a eccentrically located, pinpoint, round, basophilic nucleus (Figure 2.15d).
- Canine distemper virus is transmitted by inhalation of the virus and can be found witnin RBCs and leukocytes. It forms viral inclusions in the cytoplasm of cells that have a smooth appearing surface and can stain either pink or light blue.
- *Ehrlichia canis* is a pathogen transmitted by ticks and found within monocytes. It is a rounded, granular-appearing structure in the cytoplasm that typically stains slightly lighter purple than the monocyte nucleus.
- *Ehrlichia ewingii* is also transmitted by ticks and looks similar to *E. canis* but is found within neutrophils (Figure 2.15e).
- *Hepatozoon canis* and *Hepatozoon americanum* are large lightly basophilic oval to rectangular organisms that are observed in neutrophils and monocytes. These organisms can be transmitted by ticks.
- *Anaplasma platys* is transmitted by ticks and infects platelets. This organism forms a rounded granular structure that stains deep purple (Figure 2.15f).
- Epicellular RBC pathogens
  - *Mycoplasma haemocanis* appears similar to other *Mycoplasma* spp. It has been experimentally transmitted by ticks. It forms tiny, basophilic cocci, or rings on the edge of the erythrocyte membrane.
- Extracellular parasites
  - *Dipetalonema reconditum* is a nonpathogenic organism that is transmitted by mosquitoes. Microfilaria have a head that is the same width as the body and a long, whip-like tail that often curls up giving the organism a fish-hook appearance.
  - *Dirofilaria immitis* is transmitted by mosquitoes. It is a pathogenic organism that causes heartworm disease. Circulating microfilaria have a tapered head (compared to the body section) and a pointed tail (Figure 2.16a).
  - *Trypanosoma cruzi* is a protozoal organism that is transmitted by triatomine bugs. In the circulation, these organisms are elongated with pointed cytoplasm at their leading edge and a flagellum at their lagging edge.
- C. Blood parasites of horses
  - Intracellular RBC pathogens
    - *Babesia equi* and *Babesia caballi* are transmitted by ticks and can infect equine RBCs. They appear as small- to medium-sized piriform structures with a small amount of clear, rounded cytoplasm and a eccentrically located, pinpoint, round basophilic nucleus.
    - *Theileria* spp. are transmitted by ticks and form small piriform structures with scant, clear cytoplasm and a small, round basophilic nucleus.

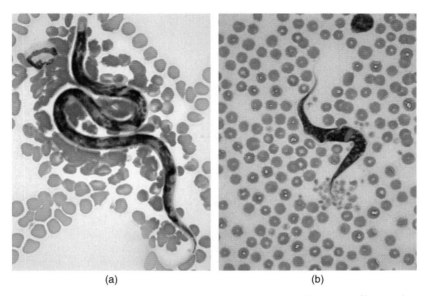

(a)   (b)

Figure 2.16   Extracellular blood parasites. (a) *Dirofilaria immitis* – extracellular microfilaria with a tapered head from a mixed-breed dog (917× magnification). (b) *Trypanosoma theileri* from a cow – an elongated protozoal organism with pointed cytoplasm at the leading edge and a flagellum at the lagging edge (approximately 917× magnification).

- Extracellular parasites
  - *Setaria equina* infestations cause minimal disease in horses, but microfilaria may be observed in the peripheral blood. This organism is transmitted by mosquitoes.
D. Blood parasites of cattle
  - Intracellular RBC pathogens
    - *Anaplasma marginale* is a small, round basophilic organism often found near the margin of an RBC membrane (Figure 2.15g). The organism is transmitted by ticks.
    - *Anaplasma centrale* is also transmitted by ticks. It is a small, round basophilic organism seen within RBCs of cattle.
    - *Babesia bovis and Babesia bigemina* are transmitted by ticks and form relatively large tear-drop-shaped structures in RBCs. These organisms have clear cytoplasm and an eccentrically located, round basophlic nucleus.
    - *Theileria* spp. form small piriform structures with scant, clear cytoplasm and a small, round basophilic nucleus. They are transmitted by ticks.
  - Epicellular RBC pathogens
    - *Mycoplasma wenyoni* appears similar to other *Mycoplasma* spp. They can be transmitted by biting insects including lice and mosquitoes. They form basophilic cocci or rings present on the edge of erythrocyte membranes.
  - Extracellular parasites
    - *Trypanosoma theileri* is a protozoal organism that typically is nonpathogenic in cattle. Circulating organisms are elongated with pointed cytoplasm at their

leading edge and a flagellum at their lagging edge (Figure 2.16b). This organism is transmitted by triatomine bugs.

Hematology Methods

A. Blood sample handling and collection

In order to accurately report data in a CBC, proper blood sample handling and collection methods must be followed strictly. Tubes must always be clearly labeled with the patient identification. If the sample is submitted to a pathologist, include the patient history as it often allows for a more definitive interpretation of the sample results.

- Whole, unclotted blood is needed to acquire CBC data.
  - EDTA is the preferred anticoagulant for mammalian blood.
  - Overnight fasting is recommended for monogastric animals (including cats and dogs) to avoid lipemia.
    - Lipemia refers to blood samples that have high concentrations of cholesterols and triglycerides.
    - Substances in lipemic samples interfere with plasma protein, fibrinogen, and Hb determination.
- It is best to collect a blood sample into a vacuum tube to reduce clot formation.
  - Clots must be avoided because they cause platelet and WBC counts to be falsely decreased.
- Vacuum collection ensures that the correct amount of blood is present to have the ideal ratio of blood and anticoagulant in the sample.
  - When blood tubes are under-filled, the PCV and Hct will be falsely decreased due to excess anticoagulant in the sample.
- Iatrogenic hemolysis (lysis of RBCs) due to poor blood collection techniques should be avoided.
  - Hemolysis interferes with determination of plasma protein, fibrinogen, and erythrocyte parameters.
- Ideally, blood samples for a CBC should be processed within 2 hours of collection.
  - If sample processing is delayed, the sample should be refrigerated.
  - 24 hours after blood collection, erythrocyte parameters and total WBC counts usually are still accurate, but platelet counts are inaccurate. In addition, it is more difficult to identify subsets of leukocytes in stored blood, so the accuracy of the WBC differential may be questionable.

B. Blood volume calculations

You can safely remove 20% of a healthy patient's blood volume during phlebotomy. It is critical to determine the amount of blood that can be collected from very small patients to avoid causing hypovolemic shock. It is helpful to know these calculations to maximize the amount of blood that can be collected from blood donors without harming the donor.

- The relative amount of blood in the body varies with species, breed, and age of the animal.
- In the clinical setting, blood collection volume calculations often are simplified to allow for more rapid determination of how much blood can be collected.
  - First, calculate the animal's weight in grams.
    - To convert pounds to kilograms, divide the weight in pounds by 2.2 lb/kg.
      - An adult dog that weighs 60 pounds has a metric weight of 60 lb ÷ 2.2 lb/kg = 27 kg.
    - To convert kilograms to grams, multiply the weight in kilograms by 1000 g/kg.
      - A 60 lb adult dog weighs 27 kg × 1000 g/kg = 27,000 g.
  - Next, estimate that the amount of blood that can safely be collected is equal to 1% of the patient's body weight.
    - 1% of 27,000 g = 270 g.
    - Estimate that the specific gravity of blood is equal to the specific gravity of water (1 mL weighs 1 g).
    - 270 g × 1 mL/g = 270 mL
  - 270 mL of blood can safely be collected from a healthy, 60 lb, adult dog.
C. PCV and total plasma protein (TP)
   The PCV and TP of a blood sample can be quickly determined without an automated hematology analyzer.
- Equipment needed
  - Two microhematocrit tubes precoated with EDTA or heparin
  - Clay
  - Microhematocrit centrifuge
  - PCV scale
  - Refractometer with a scale for protein concentration
- Procedure
  - Whole blood is collected into two microhematocrit tubes.
  - One end of each microhematocrit tube is filled with a small amount of clay to prevent leakage of blood (Figure 2.17a and b).
  - Tubes are placed in a microhematocrit centrifuge with the clay facing to the outside of the rotor.
  - The samples are centrifuged 12,000 × g for 5 minutes.
  - PCV
    - The centrifuged tube (Figure 2.17c) is lined up on a PCV scale so that the interface between the clay and the blood sample is at the 0% mark and the top of the sample (at the interface of the plasma and the air in the tube) is at the 100% mark on the scale (Figure 2.17d).
    - The line that crosses the interface between the packed cells and the plasma is traced back to the PCV scale to read the percentage of cells in the blood sample (Figure 2.17d).
    - To more closely estimate Hct, the line that crosses the interface between the packed RBCs and the buffy coat is traced back to the PCV scale to read the percentage of RBCs in the blood sample (Figure 2.17d).

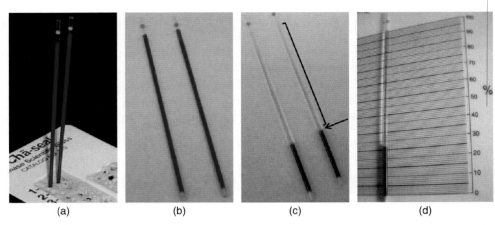

(a)   (b)   (c)   (d)

Figure 2.17   Packed cell volume measurement. (a and b) Microhematocrit tubes containing whole blood
are stopped with clay to prevent leakage. (c) A clear delineation between air (top), plasma (bracket), a buffy
coat containing WBCs and platelets (arrow), RBCs, and clay (bottom) can be seen in adequately centrifuged
microhematocrit tubes. (d) The centrifuged tube is lined up on a PCV scale so that the interface between the
clay and the RBCs is at the 0% mark and the interface of the plasma and the air is at the 100% mark. The
line that crosses the interface between the cells and plasma is the PCV of the sample. The PCV of this sample
is 28%. The line that crosses the interface between the RBCs and buffy coat is the Hct. The Hct of this
sample is 27%.

- TP
  - Break one of the centrifuged microhematocrit tubes just above the level of
    the packed cells.
  - Place the plasma onto a refractometer.
  - Visualize the line between light and shadow on the refractometer.
  - Record where the line between light and shadow crosses the scale that is
    used for protein measurement.
  - The TP protein concentration is typically reported in grams per deciliter.
D. Fibrinogen
    The plasma fibrinogen concentration may be reported along with a CBC.
    Dehydration and inflammation cause increases in fibrinogen, whereas decreases in
    fibrinogen may be observed in animals with coagulopathy. Methods for
    determining fibrinogen can be found in Chapter 3.
E. Manual RBC count
    Manual RBC counts are not typically performed. Instead, the PCV of the sample
    is determined and used to assess the RBC mass of the patient when an automated
    hematology analyzer is unavailable.
F. Manual platelet and WBC counts
    Manual WBC counts and manual platelet counts are performed using a
    hemocytometer.
- Equipment
  - Test tube
  - Scale
  - 1 litre container
  - 20–200 µL micropipette

- 200–1000 μL micropipette
- 10 μL pipette tips
- 1000 μL pipette tips
- Ammonium oxalate solution
  - 11.45 g ammonium oxalate
  - 1.0 g Sorensen's phosphate buffer
  - 0.1 g thimerosal
  - Fill to 1000 mL with purified water
- Hemocytometer (Figure 1-5a)
- Petri dish
- Absorbent paper
- Microscope with 10× and 40× objective lenses
- Sample dilution and loading
  - Mix the patient's whole blood (preferably EDTA-treated) sample by inverting the tube several times.
  - Add 1 part whole blood to 99 parts ammonium oxalate solution to lyse the RBCs and create 1:100 dilution of the sample.
    - Example: Add 10 μL of EDTA-treated blood to 990 μL of ammonium oxalate solution to achieve a 1:100 dilution.
    - RBC lysing solutions may be purchased in containers designed to fill with the correct amount of blood.
  - Mix the sample using a pipette or gently vortex the sample.
  - Incubate for 10 minutes to allow the erythrocytes to lyse.
  - Be sure that the hemocytometer is clean and the proper coverslip is in place.
  - Mix the sample using a pipette or gently vortex the sample.
  - Pipette 10 μL of the mixed sample onto each chamber of the hemocytometer (Figure 1.5b).
  - Allow the cells to settle by incubating the hemocytometer for 10 minutes in a petri dish containing a wet piece of absorbent paper (Figure 1.5c).
- WBC count
  - Calculate the average number of nucleated cells in one 1 mm grid section on the hemocytometer (Figure 2.18). See Chapter 1 for important details about how to count the cells in a hemocytometer chamber.
  - The number of nucleated cells per microliter of blood is determined using the formula:
    - (Nucleated cells/grid × dilution) ÷ 0.1 μL/grid = nucleated cells per microliter
    - Example: If the sample dilution factor is 1:100 and the average number of nucleated cells in a 1 mm grid section is 14, then (14 cells/grid × 100) ÷ 0.1 μL/grid = 14×10^3 nucleated cells/μL.
  - This is a nucleated cell count, it includes WBCs and nRBCs. This count should be corrected for any nRBCs that are present in the sample.
- Platelet count
  - Performing a manual platelet count is similar to performing a WBC count, but the number of cells in a smaller area of the hemocytometer grid is counted and the calculation of platelets per microliter is slightly different.

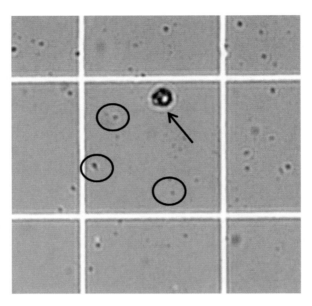

Figure 2.18   Hemocytometer grid with numerous platelets (three are circled) and one WBC (arrow).

- First determine the average number of platelets in one square of a corner 1 mm grid section on the hemocytometer (Figure 2.18).
  - Platelets in the middle of the square and touching the top and left edges of the square should be counted.
  - Do not count platelets touching the bottom and right edges of the square.
  - Note that platelet clumps will falsely lower the platelet count.
- Calculate platelets per microliter using the formula:
  - (Platelets/square × 16 squares/grid × dilution) ÷ 0.1 µL/grid = platelets/µL
  - Example: If the sample dilution factor is 1:100 and the average number of platelets in one square is 40, then (40 platelets/square × 16 squares/grid × 100) ÷ 0.1 µL/grid = 640×10^3 platelets/µL.
G. Blood smear preparation
  A blood smear should be prepared for every CBC performed to verify automated or manual cell counts and to determine cell morphology.
  - Equipment
    - Microhematocrit tubes
    - Cleaned glass slides
    - Romanowski-type stain
    - NMB stain
    - Test tubes
  - Prepare a blood smear
    - Draw a small amount of well-mixed, whole blood into a microhematocrit tube.
      - EDTA is the preferred anticoagulant.
    - Place a drop of blood onto one end of a clean slide (Figure 2.19a).

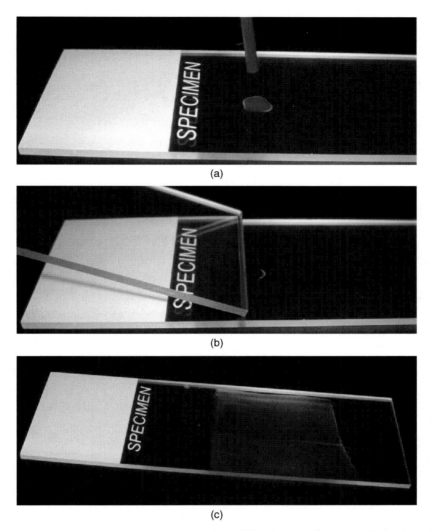

Figure 2.19   Blood smear technique. (a) A 2–3 mm drop of blood in placed on one end of a clean glass slide. (b) A second slide is placed on the blood drop to spread the blood drop across with width of the first slide. The second slide is then moved evenly down the length of the first slide to smear the blood. (c) This unstained blood smear is of the appropriate thickness to contain a cellular monolayer where cell morphology is assessed. Note that the entire blood sample remains on the first slide and creates a feathered edge where larger cells, platelet clumps, and microfilaria often are observed.

- Place a second slide onto the drop of blood (Figure 2.19b).
- Gently push (or pull) the second slide to the other end of the slide containing the sample.
  - The goal is to create a monolayer of cells without pulling any cells off of the end of the slide.

- When done correctly, the smear is smooth, nearly see-through, and has a "feathered edge" (Figure 2.19c).
  - Individual cellular morphology is examined within the monolayer using microscopy.
- Air-dry and stain the blood smear as described in Chapter 1.
  - Both Romanowski-type and NMB stains are very important for evaluation of erythrocytes.

H. Buffy coat smear preparation

   A buffy coat smear is used concentrate WBCs and platelets when counts are low so that morphology can be examined more efficiently.

- Equipment needed
  - Two microhematocrit tubes precoated with EDTA or heparin
  - Clay
  - Microhematocrit centrifuge
  - Glass cutting instrument
  - 1 cc syringe
  - Cleaned glass slides
  - Romanowski-type stain
- Procedure
  - Whole blood is collected into two microhematocrit tubes.
  - One end of each microhematocrit tube is filled with a small amount of clay to prevent leakage of blood.
  - Tubes are placed in a microhematocrit centrifuge with the clay facing to the outside of the rotor.
  - The samples are centrifuged 12,000 × g for 5 minutes.
  - WBCs and platelets that sediment to the interface between RBCs (on the bottom) and plasma (on the top) are collected.
    - A centrifuged microhematocrit tube is scored at the interface of WBCs/platelets and RBCs using a glass cutting instrument.
    - The portion of the microhematocrit tube containing RBCs is discarded.
    - Place the cut end of the microhematocrit tube over a clean glass slide so that WBCs and platelets are closest to the slide.
    - Fill a 1 cc syringe with a small amount of air.
    - Place the 1 cc syringe over the unbroken end of the microhematocrit tube and push the plunger to force air into the microhematocrit tube so that WBCs and platelets are placed onto the glass slide.
    - Place a second slide onto the drop of WBCs and platelets.
    - Gently pull a second slide to the other end of the slide containing the sample.
      - The goal is to create a monolayer of cells without pulling any cells off of the end of the slide.
      - When done correctly, the smear is smooth, nearly see-through, and has a "feathered edge."
    - Individual cellular morphology is examined within the monolayer using microscopy.
- Air-dry and stain the blood smear as described in Chapter 1.

- Romanowski-type stains are typically utilized.

I. Blood smear evaluation
  - Equipment
    - Microscope with 10× or 20×, 40× or 50×, and 100× objective lenses
    - Immersion oil
  - Be sure that the microscope condenser is raised up and the iris is open (Figure 1.2a).
  - Examine the entire blood smear at low magnification (10× or 20× objective lens).
    - Evaluate overall cellularity.
    - Determine if the RBC distribution is normal. In healthy animals, RBCs are evenly distributed throughout the monolayer of a blood smear.
    - Determine if there is platelet clumping (Figure 2.20a).
    - Check for cells that are not normally seen in peripheral blood (mast cells, blasts, etc.).
    - Look for microfilaria (Figure 2.20b).
    - It is critical to examine the feathered edge of the slide because larger cells, cell clumps, and microfilaria are often found there.
  - Estimate the WBC count.
    - Count the total number of WBCs in 10 randomly chosen microscopic fields (this can be done at low power or 40× magnification).
    - Determine the average the number of WBCs present in one field by dividing the total count by 10.
    - Multiply the average number of WBCs in one field by the power of the objective lens *squared*.
    - For example, if (on average) there are 24 WBCs in a field when examining the smear with the 20× objective lens, then there are approximately 24×20^2 cells per microliter of blood = 9600 WBCs/µL.

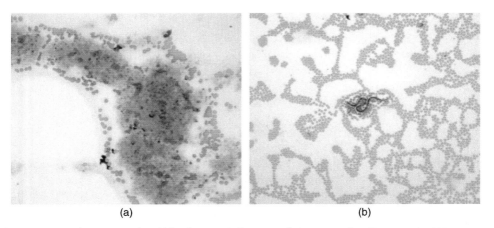

(a)   (b)

Figure 2.20   Findings in peripheral blood smears at low magnification (Wright–Giemsa stain, 200× magnification). (a) A large clump of platelets from a domestic shorthaired cat. (b) Microfilaria in a mixed-breed dog.

Table 2.3   The importance of calculating absolute cell counts.

	Case 1		Case 2		Reference Intervals	
	%	/μL	%	/μL	%	/μL
WBC count	–	5,500	–	14,000	–	5,400–14,300
Neutrophil	75	4,125	75	*10,500*	22–75	2,260–8,580
Lymphocyte	16	*880*	16	2,240	16–68	1,500–7,700
Monocyte	8	440	8	*1,120*	0–14	0–1,000
Eosinophil	1	55	1	140	0–10	0–1,000
Basophil	0	0	0	0	0–4	0–290

The total cell counts and all percentage values are within the reference intervals for both animals (Cases 1 and 2). When the absolute counts are calculated, several clinically important abnormalities are detected (in italics). Case 1 is a lymphopenic animal. Case 2 has a neutrophilia and a monocytosis.

- The more evenly distributed the cells are in the smear, the more accurate this estimation becomes.
- This estimate varies slightly with the type of microscope used.
- Determine the differential leukocyte count using a 40× or 50× objective lens. Check to see if the objective lens requires immersion oil by reading the information printed on the side of the lens.
  - The absolute number of each WBC is calculated by determining the percentage of each WBC out of 200 leukocytes on the smear and then multiplying that percentage by the total corrected WBC count.
  - It is critical to determine the absolute number of each type of leukocyte present rather than only reporting the percentage of each leukocyte observed.
    - An example of why this is important is given in Table 2.3.
  - Note that some nucleated cells may be nRBCs instead of WBCs.
    - The presence of several nRBCs will falsely elevate the WBC count. It is important to correct for this false elevation before calculating the number of different leukocytes present in the sample.
    - Some hematology analyzers automatically correct for nRBCs, others do not. Leukocyte counts determined using a hemocytometer must be corrected for nRBCs.
    - Nucleated RBCs are expressed as the number of nRBCs per 100 WBCs. The corrected WBC count = 100 × WBC count/(100 + nRBCs).
- Using the 100× objective lens and the immersion oil, evaluate cellular morphology and estimate the platelet count.
  - As previously mentioned, abnormalities in erythrocyte, leukocyte, and platelet morphology can help diagnose several disease conditions.
  - The number of platelets present per microliter of blood can be estimated if platelet clots are not present in the blood smear.
    - Determine the total number of platelets in 10 100× microscopic fields.

TECHNICIAN TIP 2–3:

Example of how to calculate the absolute cell counts of subsets of leukocytes in peripheral blood.

- You collect Lucky's blood, place it into an EDTA tube, and process the sample for a CBC.
- Lucky's blood has an average of 10 nucleated cells per 1 mm grid on the hemocytometer. So Lucky's manual WBC count = 10 × 100 ÷ 0.1 = 10,000/µL.
- Next you differentiate 200 WBCs from one another on a blood smear. Of the 200 WBCs counted, 80% are segmented neutrophils, 12% are lymphocytes, 5% are monocytes, and 3% are eosinophils.
- The blood smear contains 10 nRBCs per 100 WBCs counted.
- The corrected WBC count = 100 × WBCs/(100 + nRBCs)
  - Lucky's corrected WBC count = 100 × 10,000/(100 + 10) = 9091/µL
  - The corrected WBC count is typically rounded to two significant figures = 9100/µL
- The absolute WBC differential counts are as follows:
  - Segmented neutrophils = 9100/µL × 0.80 = 7280/µL
  - Lymphocytes = 9100/µL × 0.12 = 1092/µL
  - Monocytes = 9100/µL × 0.05 = 455/µL
  - Eosinophils = 9100/µL × 0.03 = 273/µL

- Calculate the average number of platelets per 100× field and multiply by 15,000.
- Healthy animals typically have at least 12 platelets per 100× microscopic field.

J. Reticulocyte count

A whole blood sample is stained with NMB and smeared onto a slide so that the percentage of reticulocytes in the sample can be determined. This test is not useful in horses and usually is unnecessary in cattle. Horses do not release reticulocytes into the blood stream. Any reticulocytes in the peripheral blood are considered a regenerative response in cattle and typically can be detected as polychromatophils on a peripheral blood smear. In cats and dogs, low numbers of polychromatophils are a normal finding in peripheral blood. A reticulocyte count is performed in cats and dogs to determine if reticulocytes are increased in anemic patients.

- Equipment
  - Microscope with 100× objective lens
  - Immersion oil
- Procedure
  - Prepare an NMB-stained blood smear (see above).
  - Scan the slide at a low magnification with the condenser raised up and the iris open.
  - Examine the blood smear microscopically at 100× magnification using immersion oil.
  - Determine the percentage of reticulocytes out of 1000 RBCs on the slide.

- Example: If there are 10 punctate reticulocytes (Figure 2.2c), 30 aggregate reticulocytes (Figure 2.2d), and 760 non-staining RBCs present, there are 30/1000 = 3% aggregate reticulocytes in the sample.
- Reticulocyte counts must be corrected to account for the severity of the patient's anemia.
  - A corrected reticulocyte percentage can be calculated for cats and dogs to determine if regeneration is occurring in response to an anemia.
    - Values >0.4% in the cat and >1% in the dog are considered regenerative responses.
    - Corrected reticulocyte percentage = observed reticulocyte percentage × [patient Hct (%) ÷ normal Hct (%)].
  - In place of a corrected reticulocyte percentage, an absolute reticulocyte count can be calculated by multiplying the reticulocyte percentage acquired from a slide by the RBC count acquired from an automated hematology analyzer.
    - Values >60,000 reticulocytes/µL in the cat and >80,000 reticulocytes/µL in the dog are considered regenerative.
    - Absolute reticulocyte count (/µL) = percentage of reticulocytes (as a decimal) × RBC/µL.
- Remember that a regenerative response is not observed until at least 48–72 hours after anemia occurs.

K. Saline agglutination test

   It is important to confirm that agglutination is truly occurring by performing a saline agglutination test.
- Equipment
  - 0.9% saline
  - Plastic test tubes
  - Plastic transfer pipets
  - Glass slides
  - Cover slips
  - Microscope with a 40× objective lens
- Procedure
  - Mix 1 part 0.9% saline with 1 part well-mixed whole blood in a test tube.
  - Place a drop of the mixture onto a glass slide.
  - Place a coverslip onto the sample (Figure 2.21a).
  - Allow the cells to settle under the coverslip for a few minutes.
  - Examine the sample for agglutination using the microscope with the condenser lowered.
  - If agglutination is present (Figure 2.21b), the sample is truly positive for agglutination and indicates that the patient has an IMHA.

L. Collection of blood for determination of SI or TIBC
- Equipment
  - Red-topped blood collection tube
  - Centrifuge

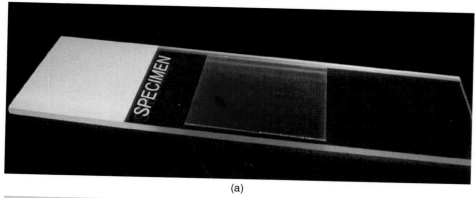

(a)

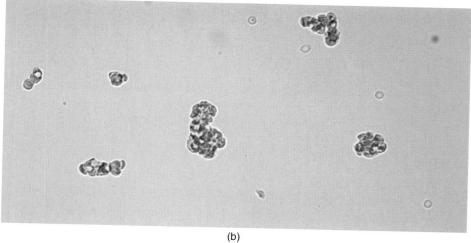

(b)

Figure 2.21   Saline agglutination test. (a) Wet-mount of a blood sample mixed 1:1 with saline. (b) Positive saline agglutination test (200× magnification, wet mount).

- Procedure
  - Blood is collected into a blood collection tube that does not contain any anticoagulant.
  - Incubate at room temperature for 15–30 minutes to allow the blood to clot.
  - Centrifuge for 10 minutes at 1000 × g to fully separate the serum from clotted blood cells.
  - Remove the serum from the blood clot and place the serum into a separate tube for measurement of iron or TIBC.
  - SI and TIBC measurements are performed using automated analyzers and testing procedures that have been validated for the appropriate species.
  - Samples being shipped to a veterinary diagnostic laboratory should be refrigerated and shipped on ice packs.

M. Crossmatching procedure
- Equipment
  - Centrifuge
  - 0.9% saline
  - Test tubes
  - Water bath or heat block
  - Microscope with a 10× objective lens
- Procedure
  - Obtain an anticoagulated blood sample in EDTA (purple-top tube) and a clotted blood sample (red-top tube) from both the patient and the donor.
  - Centrifuge the samples and separate the plasma and serum from the cell pellets. *Keep the serum* from the red-topped tubes (antibodies are there) and the cell pellets from the EDTA-treated samples.
  - Wash the cell pellets from the EDTA tubes in 0.9% saline.
    - Mix the sample pellet with 0.9% saline and centrifuge the sample for 5 minutes at $1000 \times g$.
    - Carefully remove the saline from the cell pellet.
    - Repeat three times.
  - Resuspend the cells in 0.9% saline to a dilute tomato juice color (2–4% RBC suspension).
  - Mix the following suspensions for crossmatching:
    - Major crossmatch
      - 1 drop DONOR RBC suspension
      - 2 drops PATIENT serum
    - Minor crossmatch
      - 1 drop PATIENT RBC suspension
      - 2 drops DONOR serum
    - Patient auto-control (should be negative)
      - 1 drop PATIENT RBC suspension
      - 2 drops PATIENT serum
    - Donor auto-control (should be negative)
      - 1 drop DONOR RBC suspension
      - 2 drops DONOR serum
  - Incubate the mixtures for 15–30 minutes at 37°C.
  - Centrifuge the samples (15 seconds, $1000 \times g$).
  - Macroscopic examination
    - Look for hemolysis.
      - If the animals have compatible blood types, no hemolysis will be observed.
      - If hemolysis is seen, the donor and patient are not compatible and the transfusion should not be performed.
    - Rotate the tube to look for obvious clumping of the RBCs as they come off of the cell pellet.
      - RBC clumping indicates that donor and patient are not compatible and the transfusion should not be performed.
      - If RBCs do not clump, the sample should be examined microscopically.

- Microscopic examination
  - Mix the sample and place a drop onto a slide.
  - Lower the microscope condenser and examine the sample.
  - No agglutination will be seen if animals have compatible blood types.
  - An incompatible sample will have agglutination (Figure 2.21b).
N. Coombs' test

The Coombs' test is a direct antiglobulin test. Species-specific reagents are needed to perform this test.

- Equipment
  - Centrifuge
  - 0.9% saline
  - Test tubes
  - Species-specific Coombs' test kit
- Procedure
  - Mix EDTA-treated whole blood with 0.9% saline to produce a dilute tomato juice color (2–4% RBC suspension).
  - Place two drops of the RBC suspension into a separate test tube.
  - Centrifuge the sample for 5 minutes at 1000 × g.
  - Remove the excess supernatant and wash the cell pellet in 0.9% saline.
    - To wash the cell pellet, mix the sample pellet with 0.9% saline and centrifuge the sample for 5 minutes at 1000 × g.
    - Carefully remove the saline from the cell pellet.
    - Repeat three times.
  - Incubate the cells with species–specific antiglobulin reagent and centrifuge the sample per the directions in the Coombs' test kit.
  - Macroscopic examination
    - Rotate the tube to look for obvious clumping of the RBCs as they come off of the cell pellet.
      - RBC clumping is a positive result and suggests that the animal has an IMHA.
      - If RBCs do not clump, the sample should be examined microscopically.
  - Microscopic examination
    - Mix the sample and place a drop onto a slide for microscopic examination.
      - RBC clumping is a positive result and suggests that the animal has an IMHA (Figure 2.21b).
      - If no RBC clumping is observed, record a negative Coombs' test result.

Further Reading

Giger U. (2000) Regenerative anemias caused by blood loss or hemolysis. In: S.J. Ettinger & E.C. Feldman (eds.) *Textbook of Veterinary Internal Medicine* (5th ed.) pp.1801-1802). Philadelphia, PA: WB Saunders Company.

Greenhalgh J.F., Aitken J.N., & Gunn J.B. (1972). Kale anaemia: A survey of kale feeding practices and anaemia in cattle on dairy farms in England and Scotland. *Research in Veterinary Science*, 13(1):15–21.

Harvey, J.W. (ed) (2012) *Veterinary Hematology: A Diagnostic Guide and Color Atlas.* Elsevier Saunders, St. Louis, MO.

Houston D.M. & Myers S.L. (1993). A review of Heinz-body anemia in the dog induced by toxins. *Veterinary & Human Toxicology,* 35(2):158–161.

Jain, N.C. (ed) (1993) *Essentials of Veterinary Hematology.* Lea & Febiger, Philadelphia, PA.

Maxwell A.P., Lappin T.R.J., Johnston C.F., Bridges J.M. & McGeown M.G. (1990). Erythropoietin production in kidney tubular cells. *British Jourinal of Hematology,* 74:535–539.

Meintker L., Ringwald J., Rauh M. & Krause S.W. (2013). Comparison of automated differential blood cell counts from Abbott Sapphire, Siemens Advia 120, Beckman Coulter DxH 800, and Sysmex XE-2100 in normal and pathologic samples. *American Journal of Clinical Pathology,* 139(5):641–650.

Morris J.G., Cripe W.S., Chapman H.L. Jr,, *et al.* (1984). Selenium deficiency in cattle associated with Heinz bodies and anemia. *Science,* 223(4635):491–493.

Vacha J. (1983). Red cell lifespan. N.S. Agar & P.G. Board (eds.) *Red Blood Cells of Domestic Mammals,* p. 67. New York, NY: Elsevier.

Weinstein, N.M., Blais, M.C., Harris, K., Oakley, D.A., Aronson, L.R. & Giger, U. (2007). A newly recognized blood group in domestic shorthair cats: the Mik red cell antigen. *Journal of Veterinary Internal Medicine,* 21: 287–292.

Weiss D.J. & Wardrop K.J. (eds.) (2010). *Schalm's Veterinary Hematology* (6th ed.). Ames, IA: Wiley-Blackwell.

Weiss D.J., McClay C.B., Christopher M.M., Murphy M. & Perman V. (1990). Effects of propylene glycol-containing diets on acetaminophen-induced methemoglobinemia in cats. *Journal of the American Veterinary Medical Association,* 196:1816–1819.

Whitelaw D.M. & Bell M. (1966). The intravascular lifespan of monocytes. *Blood,* 28:455–464.

Interpretation and comments for Case 1

Interpretation: The patient has a macrocytic, hypochromic anemia as indicated by the decreased Hct, Hgb, and RBC with an increased MCV and decreased MCHC. The absolute reticulocyte count is $0.045 \times (3.3 \times 10^6/\mu L) = 148,500/\mu L$, which indicates a regenerative response to the anemia. Spherocytes were detected and are highly suggestive of immune-mediated hemolytic anemia. There is a leukocytosis composed of a neutrophilia, lymphopenia, and monocytosis. This combination is consistent with inflammation and stress. The thrombocytopenia is concerning and may indicate increased platelet consumption or destruction.

Comment: Additional diagnostic testing is warranted in this case. A Coombs' test could help confirm the suspicion of immune-mediated disease. Underlying causes of immune-mediated disease should be tested for. Assessment of the coagulation pathway is highly recommended.

Interpretation and comments For Case 2

Interpretation: This patient has an erythrocytosis as indicated by the increased PCV, Hgb, and RBC. Given the physical examination findings the most likely cause of the hemoconcentration is dehydration. The leukocytosis with a neutrophilia and left shift indicates that this is an inflammatory leukogram and the lymphopenia suggests that there is a concurrent stress response. Both dehydration and inflammation can contribute to the increased fibrinogen concentration.

Comment: The inflammatory response and the diarrhea are likely linked to the same underlying disease. Further diagnostics to determine if there is an infectious cause of diarrhea are recommended.

Interpretation and comments for Case 3

Interpretation: This animal has a normocytic, normochromic anemia as indicated by the decreased Hct, Hgb, and RBC with a normal MCV and MCHC. The anemia is likely nonregenerative because no polychromasia or anisocytosis was observed. Keratocytes are present suggestive of oxidative damage to the red blood cells. Echinocytes are frequently due to improper drying of the slide during preparation of the blood smear. The leukocyte count is within the reference interval, but there is a neutropenia and a left shift indicating that this patient is having difficulty keeping up with an inflammatory process. The thrombon is within the reference interval.

Comment: Close examination of the patient to determine the cause of the inflammation is critical.

Activities

Multiple Choice Questions

1. Which of the following components of blood is present in plasma but *not* in serum?
   A) Albumin
   B) Gamma-globulin
   C) Hormones
   D) Fibrinogen

2. A major crossmatch tests for which of the following interactions?
   A) Patient antibodies that cause donor RBCs to lyse/agglutinate
   B) Donor antibodies that cause patient RBCs to lyse/agglutinate
   C) Patient antibodies that cause patient RBCs lyse/agglutinate
   D) Donor antibodies that cause donor RBCs lyse/agglutinate

3. True or false. The term for increased numbers of neutrophil bands is a "left shift."

4. True or false. If a small blood clot is present in a purple-topped tube, the sample can be processed for a CBC once the clot has been removed.

5. True or false. Giant platelets are observed frequently in blood smears of healthy cats.

Hemostasis

chapter

3

Amy L. MacNeill
Colorado State University,
Fort Collins, CO, USA

Learning Objectives

1. Become familiar with key proteins and cellular components involved in hemostasis.
2. Estimate the platelet count in a peripheral blood sample.
3. Calculate plasma fibrinogen concentration.
4. Measure buccal mucosal bleeding time.
5. Determine activated clotting time.
6. Learn blood collection and storage methods for analysis of coagulation pathways.
   - Prothrombin time
   - Activated partial thromboplastin time
7. Know blood collection and storage methods for analysis of fibrinolysis.
   - Fibrin degradation products
   - D-dimer
   - Antithrombin III
8. Understand blood collection and storage methods for specialized platelet function tests.
   - Clot retraction
   - Platelet aggregation assays
   - Thromboelastography

KEY TERMS

Hemostasis
Platelet
Coagulation
Fibrinolysis

Clinical Pathology and Laboratory Techniques for Veterinary Technicians, First Edition.
Edited by Anne Barger and Amy MacNeill.
© 2015 John Wiley & Sons, Inc. Published 2015 by John Wiley & Sons, Inc.
Companion Website: www.wiley.com/go/barger/vettechclinpath

Case example 1

Signalment: 10 year-old, intact, female, mixed-breed dog. History: Mammary gland adeno-carcinoma diagnosed 1 year ago. Has had 2 radical mastectomies. Physical exam: clinically dehydrated; pale, yellow, and tacky mucous membranes. Plan: Blood was drawn and placed into a purple-topped tube to collect whole blood for a CBC. After results were obtained, additional blood was collected into a blue-topped tube for analysis of coagulation data.

CBC

Parameter	Result	Reference Range
Hct	15%	35.0–57.0
Hgb	4.5 g/dL	11.9–18.9
RBC	$3.3 \times 10^6/\mu L$	$4.95–7.87 \times 10^6$
MCV	78 fL	60.0–77.0
MCHC	30 g/dL	32.0–36.3
Reticulocytes (uncorrected)	4.5%	
WBC	17,700/μL	6,000–17,000
Segmented Neutrophils	15,753/μL	3,000–11,500
Lymphocytes	531/μL	1,000–4,800
Monocytes	1,416/μL	150–1,350
Eosinophils	0/μL	100–1,250
Basophils	0/μL	0–100
Platelets	48,000/μL	200,000–600,000
RBC morphology	1+ spherocytes	

Coagulation panel

Test	Result	Reference Range
PT	>60 seconds	6–10
PTT	>60 seconds	6–16
FDP	>40 ng/mL	<10

Case example 2

Signalment: 2-year-old, castrated, male, domestic short-haired cat. History: Indoor/outdoor cat. Physical examination: The cat is weak and has pale mucous membranes, bilateral epis-taxis, and a grade II/VI heart murmur. Plan: Blood was collected into a tube containing diatomaceous earth and a blue-topped tube for a coagulation panel.

Coagulation panel

Test	Result	Reference Range
PT	>50 seconds	6–10
PTT	>30 seconds	6–16
ACT	>200 seconds	<165

Case example 3

Signalment: 8-month-old, female, Doberman pincher. History: Healthy per owner. The animal is at the veterinary clinic to have an ovariohysterectomy. Physical examination: No abnormalities. Plan: Discuss potential bleeding complications with the owner and perform a BMBT before spaying. Results: BMBT > 5 minutes.

Introduction

Hemostasis prevents the loss of blood through blood vessels that have been damaged during illness or injury. The body achieves hemostasis through complex cascades of protein and cellular interactions that lead to vasoconstriction, *platelet* activation, clot formation (*coagulation*), clot resolution (*fibrinolysis*), and wound healing.

In health, most proteins involved in hemostasis exist as inactive precursors. When blood vessels are damaged, signals from the damaged cells cleave inactive coagulation factors into active proteinases. Proteinases then activate other factors until hemostasis is achieved. In addition to the coagulation factors, several cell types contribute to hemostasis including endothelial cells, platelets, and fibroblasts.

Deficiencies or dysfunctions in key factors or cellular components involved in hemostasis are not uncommon. The laboratory tests used to identify these deficiencies are the focus of this chapter.

Physiology

There are three major events that occur before a blood clot forms and hemostasis is achieved.

1. Blood vessels are damaged.
2. Blood flow is interrupted.
3. Coagulation is initiated.

The importance of these events was recognized in the late 1800s and together they are known as Virchow's Triad.

A. Platelet activation

Activation of platelets is required for blood clot formation and hemostasis. This process is a component of primary hemostasis. An accurate platelet count is an important diagnostic test to evaluate in animals with bleeding abnormalities.

- A decreased platelet count (thrombocytopenia) or defects in platelet functions often lead to the formation of multiple small hemorrhages observed in the skin. Pinpoint hemorrhages in the skin are called petechiae (Figure 3.1). Hemorrhages in the skin larger than 1 cm in diameter are called ecchymoses (Figure 3.2).
- Mammalian platelets are small fragments of cytoplasm derived from megakaryocytes.
  - Megakaryocytes are large cells that are present in hematopoietic tissues, such as the bone marrow (Figure 2.11).
  - Platelet production is stimulated by the growth factor thrombopoietin.
- Platelets have glycoproteins (GPs) on their surface that interact with other components of the coagulation system.
  - If platelet GPs are abnormal, as observed with some genetic diseases, hemostasis cannot be achieved and excessive bleeding can occur.
- Platelets contain α-granules and dense granules that store important proteins involved in coagulation.
- Examples of these proteins include Factor V, von Willebrand factor (vWF), fibrinogen, and fibronectin.

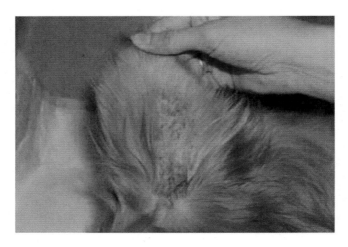

Figure 3.1   Petechiae. Pinpoint petechial hemorrhages on the ear pinna of a golden retriever.

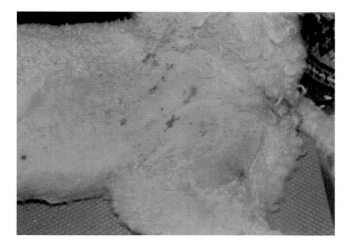

Figure 3.2   Ecchymoses. Multiple 1–2 cm ecchymotic hemorrhages on the abdomen of a poodle.

- Platelet aggregation is needed for blood clot formation.
  - Platelet aggregation requires secretion of adenosine diphosphate (ADP) and thromboxane A_2 by activated platelets. Thromboxane A_2 stimulates vasoconstriction and activates additional platelets.
  - Platelets aggregate and adhere to vWF on damaged endothelial cells via platelet glycoprotein Ib (GPIb).
- Platelet disorders may be acquired or congenital.
- Immune-mediated thrombocytopenia (ITP) is an example of a disease process that causes an acquired platelet defect due to platelet destruction.
  - Animals are thrombocytopenic.
  - Close examination of a blood smear for the presence of intracellular organisms is highly recommended (see Chapter 2).
  - Causes of ITP include infection, inflammation, drug reactions, toxins, neoplasia, and autoimmune disease.
- Disseminated intravascular coagulation (DIC) and vasculitis can lead to acquired platelet defects because of increased platelet consumption.
  - Acquired platelet defects due to decreased platelet production are often associated with bone marrow damage.
  - There are many acquired platelet defects that lead to bleeding disorders because they decrease platelet function. Relatively common examples of this are given in the following list.
    - Aspirin and other non-steroidal anti-inflammatory drugs (NSAIDs) inhibit the production thromboxane A_2 that inhibits platelet aggregation.
    - Animals with severe kidney disease (uremia) have high levels of toxic metabolites in the blood that impair platelet adhesion to endothelial cells.
    - There also are congenital defects in platelet functions and coagulation factors. Examples include von Willebrand disease (vWD) and Glanzmann's thrombasthenia.

- vWD is a relatively common congenital disorder in which animals have a decreased amount of vWF.
  - Several species, including cats and dogs, can be affected. Doberman Pinschers have a high prevalence of this disease.
  - Animals with vWD will bleed for prolonged periods of time following injury or surgery. Post-operative blood transfusion may be necessary.
- Glanzmann's thrombasthenia is caused by dysfunction of platelet glycoprotein GPIIb/IIIa.
  - Without functional GPIIb/IIIa, platelets cannot bind to fibrinogen normally, which prevents effective platelet aggregation and clot formation.
- The web site www.vetgen.com has information about genetic tests that are available for animals.

B. Coagulation
  - Damaged endothelial cells and activated platelets help to trigger coagulation cascades that allow blood clots to form. This process is termed secondary hemostasis. Coagulation abnormalities may cause hemorrhaging and hematoma formation.
  - Coagulation cascades are separated into the intrinsic pathway and the extrinsic pathway, which converge into the common pathway and lead to clot formation (Figure 3.3). These coagulation pathways are complex and include extensive feedback loops that enable newly activated factors to affect the activation of earlier components in the cascades. Activated coagulation factors are designated by placing a lowercase letter "a" after the name of the factor.
  - The coagulation pathways described in the following list do not account for every molecule that plays a role in coagulation; the importance of proteins released by platelets, endothelial cells, and fibroblasts should not be overlooked. Nevertheless, grouping coagulation factors into separate pathways is useful because abnormalities in the different pathways correspond to different diagnostic test results (Figure 3.4).
    - Intrinsic coagulation is initiated when inactive precursor proteins in the plasma become bound to damaged endothelial cells. Molecules involved in this pathway include the following:
      - High-molecular-weight kininogen (HMWK)
      - Kallikrein
        - Bradykinin (which mediates pain)
      - Factor XII
      - Factor XI
      - Factor IX
        - Factor IX production is dependent on vitamin K.
      - Factor VIII
        - In the circulation, Factor VIII is complexed to (vWF).
        - vWF is required for optimal platelet adhesion damaged vessels.
      - Calcium ion (Ca^{2+}; Factor IV)
    - Extrinsic coagulation is initiated by Factor IIIa release from damaged endothelial cells. This pathway is also triggered by inflammatory mediators,

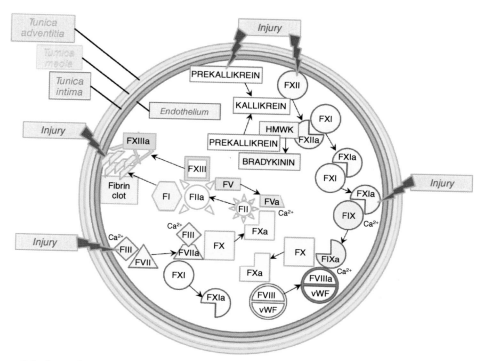

Figure 3.3   Secondary hemostasis within a blood vessel. Vascular injury causes the release of phospholipids from damaged endothelial cell membranes and triggers expression of proteins that promote coagulation. Hemostasis occurs following activation of several coagulation factors that lead to the formation of a fibrin clot. Fibrin clot formation minimizes leakage of plasma and blood cells through the damaged vessel and promotes tissue repair. Coagulation factors in this diagram are designated by the letter "F" followed by a Roman numeral. Activated coagulation factors are indicated by a lower case "a." Factors and proteins involved in the intrinsic coagulation pathway are outlined in blue. Extrinsic coagulation factors are outlined in purple. Coagulation factors of the common pathway are outlined in orange.

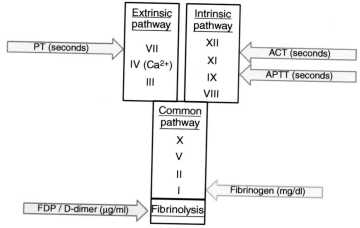

Figure 3.4   Coagulation pathway summary. Coagulation factors that contribute to extrinsic, intrinsic, and common coagulation pathways are indicated by roman numerals. The relationship of the coagulation pathways to selected diagnostic tests is shown.

bacterial endotoxins, and some coagulation factors. Components of this cascade include the following:
- Factor III (tissue factor)
- Calcium ion (Ca^{2+}; Factor IV)
- Factor VII
  - Factor VII production is dependent on vitamin K.
- The common pathway of coagulation begins with Factor X. Components of this pathway include the following:
  - Factor X
    - Factor X production is dependent on vitamin K.
  - Factor V
  - Factor II (thrombin)
    - Factor II production is dependent on vitamin K.
  - Factor I (fibrinogen)
    - Factor IIa cleaves Factor I (fibrinogen) to form fibrin.
    - Fibrin molecules bind together (polymerize) to create the scaffold for clot formation.
  - Calcium ion (Ca^{2+}; Factor IV)
  - Factor XIII
    - Factor XIIIa increases the strength of the chemical bonds between fibrin molecules and helps the clot retract.

C. Fibrinolysis
   Blood clots cannot remain in blood vessels without inhibiting blood flow to tissues and causing organ damage. The body counteracts clot formation by limiting and breaking down fibrin scaffolds. This process is called fibrinolysis (Figure 3.5).
- In health, fibrinolysis is inhibited by plasma proteins that degrade the fibrinolytic enzymes in plasma.
- When tissues are injured, tissue plasminogen activator (tPA) is protected from degradation. This allows plasminogen in the peripheral blood to be cleaved by tPA and form plasmin.
- Plasmin binds to fibrin and restricts the size of the clot that is formed during coagulation.
  - Fibrin degradation products (FDPs) and D-dimers are formed during this process.
- FDPs inhibit thrombin activation and fibrin polymerization.
- Protein C and Protein S are GPs that are important for fibrinolysis.
- The formation of Protein C and Protein S is dependent on vitamin K.
- Antithrombin III inhibits the intrinsic and common coagulation pathways by disabling thrombin and Factors IXa, Xa, XIa, and XIIa.

D. Coagulopathy
   Diseases that impair the ability of the coagulation cascade to form blood clots are coagulopathies. Acquired coagulopathies are seen more commonly than hereditary coagulopathies. Hereditary coagulopathies, such as hemophilia, are associated with decreased production of a specific coagulation factor. Acquired coagulopathies may be caused by organ dysfunction, toxicity, infection, neoplasia, and nearly every other disease process. A few common disease processes that cause coagulopathies are listed to below.
- Liver disease

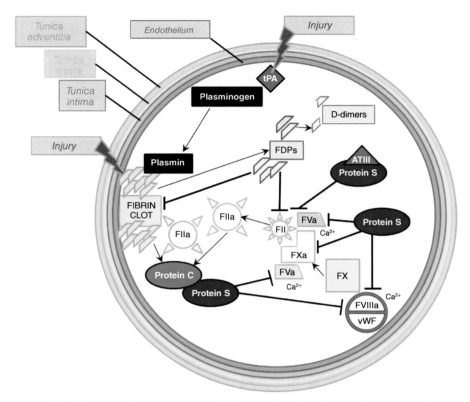

Figure 3.5   Fibrinolysis. Vascular injury causes stabilization of tPA that cleaves plasminogen to form plasmin. Plasmin breaks down fibrin clots to form fibrin degradation products (FDPs) that further degrade to form D-dimers. FDPs limit Factor II (thrombin) activation and clot formation. Protein C and Protein S are vitamin K-dependent proteins that also inhibit activation of coagulation factors and clot formation. Protein C is activated by high concentrations of thrombin and fibrin and forms a complex with Protein S in the plasma. Antithrombin III (ATIII) interacts with fibrinolytic proteins to inhibit thrombin activation. ATIII also inhibits the function of Factors IIa, IXa, Xa, XIa, and XIIa (not shown).

- Most coagulation factors are synthesized by the liver. Rarely, severe liver disease, often resulting in liver failure, causes deficiencies of coagulation factors that lead to clinical signs of bleeding.
- Vitamin K deficiency
  - The production of coagulation Factors II, VII, IX, and X requires adequate levels of vitamin K.
  - Deficiency may be caused by decreased gastrointestinal absorption of vitamin K. More commonly, vitamin K deficiency in cats and dogs is caused by coumarin (warfarin and brodifacoum) toxicity resulting in vitamin K antagonism. This is why ingestion of rat poisons containing coumarin or related rodenticides will lead to a coagulopathy.
  - Clinical signs include weakness, pallor, hypovolemia, dyspnea, epistaxis, hematuria, melena, external hematomas, hemarthrosis, and bleeding into body cavities.
  - Diagnostic abnormalities

- PT, APTT, and ACT are increased.
- Disseminated intravascular coagulopathy (DIC) leads to platelet consumption and abnormalities in the coagulation cascade.
  - Clotting is triggered throughout the vasculature system resulting in the formation of microthrombi that cause ischemia and lead to organ dysfunction. Excessive clot formation results in activation, utilization, and destruction of platelets. Thrombocytopenia often is seen and hemorrhage occurs.
  - Simultaneously, activation of the fibrinolytic system occurs. This enhances fibrin degradation and increases FDPs and D-dimers in the blood. Fibrinolysis also stimulates inflammation resulting in vasodilation, vascular stasis, and additional vascular injury and hemorrhage.
  - To diagnose DIC, at least three of the four laboratory abnormalities in the following list must be present.
    - Prolonged PT
    - Prolonged APTT
    - Increased FDPs or D-dimers
    - Decreased platelet count
  - Other test abnormalities: increased TCT, decreased fibrinogen, decreased ATIII, and schistocytes on the blood smear.

Diagnostic Testing

A. Blood collection
  - Remember the importance of blood collection methodology (Chapter 2). Traumatic venipuncture during collection of blood will cause errors in coagulation tests.
  - Platelets are easily activated during phlebotomy and should be avoided by practicing atraumatic techniques.
  - Preferably, blood is collected into a vacuum tube to reduce clot formation and ensure that the ideal ratio of blood and anticoagulant is present.
  - Overnight fasting is recommended.
  - Iatrogenic hemolysis should be avoided.

TECHNICIAN TIP 3–1: BLOOD COLLECTION METHODS FOR HEMOSTASIS TESTING

- Blood must be collected into tubes that contain an anticoagulant for most tests that evaluate hemostasis.
- Atraumatic venipuncture is necessary to prevent platelet activation.
  - Draw blood cleanly into a plastic syringe.
  - Transfer the blood into a collection tube containing anticoagulant.
  - Avoid turbulence.

B. Fibrinogen
  - Necessary for primary hemostasis (platelet aggregation)

- Fibrinogen is also a positive acute-phase protein and so its concentration increases during inflammation.
- Several methods can be used to determine plasma fibrinogen concentration. Two of these methods are described to below.
  - Heat precipitation method
  - Not discriminatory at low fibrinogen concentrations
    - Equipment needed
      - Two microhematocrit tubes precoated with ethylenediaminetetraacetate (EDTA) or heparin
      - Clay
      - Microhematocrit centrifuge
      - Refractometer with a scale for protein concentration
      - 56°C water bath or heat block
    - Procedure
      - Whole blood is collected into two microhematocrit tubes.
      - One end of each microhematocrit tube is filled with a small amount of clay to prevent leakage of blood.
      - Tubes are placed in a microhematocrit centrifuge with the clay facing to the outside of the rotor.
      - The samples are centrifuged 12,000 × g for 5 minutes.
      - One centrifuged tube is incubated at 56°C for 3 minutes to precipitate fibrinogen out of the plasma.
      - Using the other tube, the total plasma protein of the sample is measured by breaking the tube just above the level of the packed cells and then placing the plasma onto a refractometer (see Chapter 2). The total plasma protein concentration is typically reported in grams per deciliter.
      - Next, the plasma protein (g/dL) in the incubated sample is measured by breaking the tube above the level of the packed cells and placing the plasma onto a refractometer.
      - The protein concentration in the incubated sample is subtracted from the total plasma protein in the unincubated sample. This value is the fibrinogen concentration of the patient's plasma and is typically converted from grams per deciliter to milligrams per deciliter before it is reported.
      - Normal fibrinogen concentrations are typically less than 300 mg/dL.
- Clauss method
  - Equipment needed
    - Analyzer that measures fibrinogen
    - Blue-topped tube containing 3.2% sodium citrate
    - Active thrombin reagent (be sure that this reagent is not expired)
    - Centrifuge
  - Procedure
    - An analyzer designed to detect fibrinogen is required for this assay. Samples should be processed according to analyzer manufacturer instructions.
    - A small amount of citrated whole blood is added to the appropriate amount of thrombin reagent.

- Thrombin causes the fibrinogen to clot (forming fibrin) and thrombin clotting time (TCT) is recorded. TCT varies significantly between different species.
- TCT is converted mathematically into fibrinogen concentration using species-specific calculations.

C. Platelet count
  - See Chapter 2.
D. Buccal mucosal bleeding time (BMBT)
  - Used to evaluate platelet function
    - Indicative of primary hemostasis
  - Assesses platelet function
  - Equipment needed
    - Timer
    - Spring-loaded cassette
      - Allows for precise depth and length of the cut.
      - Different sizes are used in cats and dogs.
      - Animals may need to be sedated.
  - Procedure
    - Raise the lip behind an upper canine to expose the buccal mucosa.
      - The lip must remain raised away from the test site for the entire procedure.
      - The animal must not lick at the test site until the entire procedure is completed.
      - This may be easiest to do with the animal in lateral recumbency.
    - Blot the mucosa dry with a gauze pad.
    - Press the cassette flat against the mucosa.
      - Avoid any visible large vessels.
    - Firmly depress the button on the cassette to push the blade into the mucosa.
      - The blade will automatically retract back into the cassette after the mucosa has been cut.
    - Remove the cassette from the mucosal surface.
      - Begin timing immediately after removing the cassette from the mucosa.
    - Determine how long it takes for the animal to stop bleeding.
      - The length of time that it takes for the animal to stop bleeding is the BMBT.
      - Typically, bleeding stops within 3 minutes in cats and 4 minutes in dogs.
E. Clot retraction
  - Assesses platelet function
  - Not useful for patients on medications such as aspirin or thrombocytopenic patients with platelet counts less than 100,000 platelets per microliter.
  - There are simplistic clot retraction assays that are not often utilized any more (adapted from http://www.pathology.vcu.edu/education/PathLab/pages/hemostasis/cotests/clotretraction and http://mghlabtest.partners.org/coagbook/CO001000.htm accessed on December 14, 2012).
  - Collect 1–2 mL of whole blood into a red top tube.
  - Incubate the blood at 37°C.
  - Examine the sample at 1, 2, 4, and 24 hours for clot retraction.

- Clot retraction has occurred when the clot pulls away from the walls of the tube.
- The clot should retract within 1–2 hours of incubation.
- The clot should remain stable at the 24 hour time point.
- Clot lysis typically begins to occur 72 hours after blood collection.
- More precise clot retraction assays require skilled preparation of platelets and the addition of purified reagents including fibrinogen and thrombin.

F. Platelet aggregation assays
  - Specialized platelet function tests that typically must be read within 4 hours of blood collection
  - Requires an aggregometer
    - The procedure recommended by the manufacturer of the aggregometer should be followed.
  - Example procedure
    - Collect blood into a citrated tube (9 parts blood: 1 part 3.2% sodium citrate) and store at room temperature until the test is performed.
    - Isolate platelet-rich plasma by centrifuging the sample at 20°C and 150 × g for 10–15 minutes.
    - Separate the platelet-rich plasma from the pelleted red and white blood cells by pipetting the plasma into a plastic tube.
    - Add an appropriate amount of platelet agonist to the platelet-rich plasma.
      - This will activate the platelets.
      - Platelet agonists include collagen, thrombin, thromboxane A2, adenosine diphosphate, and epinephrine.
    - The change in optical density that occurs in the sample when the platelets are activated is recorded by the aggregometer.
    - The rate of platelet aggregation is calculated from the aggregometer tracing.

G. Activated clotting time (ACT)
  - Assesses intrinsic and common coagulation pathways
  - Equipment needed
    - Timer
    - Blood collection tube containing diatomaceous earth or similar particulate material (ACT tube)
    - 37°C water bath or heat block
  - Procedure
    - Blood is collected into a prewarmed tube, mixed well, and maintained at 37°C until the sample clots.
    - Two milliliter of blood is required for most blood collection tubes used to determine ACT.
    - The time it takes for the clot to form is the ACT.
    - The ACT in healthy animals should be less than 95 seconds for dogs and less than 165 seconds for cats.

H. Activated partial thromboplastin time (APTT or partial thromboplastin time, PTT)
  - Assesses intrinsic and common coagulation pathways
  - Equipment needed
    - Analyzer that measures APTT

- Blue-topped tube containing 3.2% sodium citrate
- Citrated blood from a healthy animal to be used as a control sample
- Centrifuge
- Procedure
  - Isolate plasma
    - Collect blood into a citrated tube (9 parts blood: 1 part 3.2% sodium citrate) and mix.
    - Centrifuge at $1500 \times g$ for 10–15 minutes.
    - Separate the plasma from the cell pellet by transferring the platelet-poor plasma to a plastic tube using a plastic pipette. The plasma should be used within an hour but can be refrigerated for approximately 6 hours before the test is run.
  - Analyze the plasma according to the analyzer manufacturer instructions.
    - The analyzer maintains the sample at 37°C.
    - Phospholipid, a contact activator, and calcium are added to the sample.
    - The time it takes for the clot to form is the APTT, which is measured in seconds.
  - American Labor/Lab A.C.M. Inc., Bio/Data Corporation, Diagnostica Stago Inc., Iddexx Laboratories, LAbor BioMedical Technologies GmbH, and Siemens Healthcare Diagnostics are a few of the companies that produce APTT analyzers.
  - APTT is prolonged if the patient's APTT is >30% longer than the control's APTT.
I. Prothrombin time (PT)
  - Assesses extrinsic and common coagulation pathways
  - Equipment needed
    - Analyzer that measures PT
    - Blue-topped tube containing 3.2% sodium citrate
    - Citrated blood from a healthy animal to be used as a control sample
    - Centrifuge
  - Procedure
    - Isolate plasma
    - Collect blood into a citrated tube (9 parts blood: 1 part 3.2% sodium citrate) and mix.
    - Centrifuge at $1500 \times g$ for 10–15 minutes.
    - Separate the plasma from the cells by transferring the platelet-poor plasma to a plastic tube using a plastic pipette. The plasma should be used within an hour but can be refrigerated for approximately 6 hours before the test is run.
    - Analyze the plasma according to the analyzer manufacturer instructions.
      - The analyzer maintains the sample at 37°C.
      - Calcium is added to overcome the effect of the citrate, allowing the blood to clot.
      - Tissue factor is added to the sample.
      - The time it takes for the clot to form is the PT, measured in seconds.
    - American Labor/Lab A.C.M. Inc., Bio/Data Corporation, Diagnostica Stago Inc., Iddexx Laboratories, LAbor BioMedical Technologies GmbH, and

Siemens Healthcare Diagnostics are a few of the companies that produce PT analyzers.
- PT is prolonged if the patient's PT is > 30% longer than the control's PT.

J. FDPs
- Assesses ongoing fibrinolysis
- Equipment needed
  - Blue-topped tube containing 3.2% sodium citrate
  - Antibody-based kit that detects breakdown products of fibrin
  - Centrifuge
- Procedure
- Isolate plasma
  - Collect blood into a citrated tube (9 parts blood: 1 part 3.2% sodium citrate) and mix.
  - Centrifuge at 1500 × g for 10–15 minutes.
  - Separate the plasma from the cell pellet by transferring the platelet-poor plasma to a plastic tube using a plastic pipette. Ideally, the plasma should be used within an hour.
- Analyze the plasma according to the kit manufacturer instructions.
- These tests use a monoclonal antibody to detect FDPs.
  - Latex particles coated with anti-FDP antibodies are mixed with the patient's plasma.
  - If FDPs are present, the beads agglutinate and can be seen.
  - The amount of agglutination is translated into the concentration of FDPs in the sample.
- In healthy animals, the FDP concentration is typically less than 5 µg/mL.

K. D-dimers
- Assesses fibrinolysis
- Equipment needed
  - Blue-topped tube containing 3.2% sodium citrate
  - Antibody-based kit that detects D-dimers
  - Centrifuge
- Procedure
  - Isolate plasma
    - Collect blood into a citrated tube (9 parts blood: 1 part 3.2% sodium citrate) and mix.
    - Centrifuge at 1500 × g for 10–15 minutes.
    - Separate the plasma from the cell pellet by transferring the platelet-poor plasma to a plastic tube using a plastic pipette. The plasma can be refrigerated for up to one month before the test is run.
  - Analyze the plasma according to the kit manufacturer instructions.
    - These tests use a monoclonal antibody to detect D-dimers, a specific breakdown product of fibrin.

L. Anthrombin III (ATIII)
- Increased in hypercoagulable states
- Equipment needed
  - Analyzer designed to measure ATIII

- Blue-topped tube containing 3.2% sodium citrate
- Centrifuge
- Procedure
  - Isolate plasma
    - Collect blood into a citrated tube (9 parts blood: 1 part 3.2% sodium citrate) and mix.
    - Centrifuge at $1500 \times g$ for 10–15 minutes.
    - Separate the plasma from the cell pellet by transferring the platelet-poor plasma to a plastic tube using a plastic pipette. The plasma should be used within an hour but can be refrigerated for 96 hours before the test is run.
  - Analyze the plasma according to the analyzer manufacturer instructions.
  - A chromogenic assay often is used. Chromogenic assays detect a color change when a specific chemical reaction occurs in a test sample. The substance in the test sample that causes the color change when the reaction occurs is called a chromagen.
    - A known amount of Factor IIa or Factor Xa and excess heparin and a chromogen are added to a control sample and the patient's plasma sample.
    - ATIII in the samples reacts with the coagulation factor.
    - Coagulation factor molecules that are not reacting with ATIII can react with the chromogen, causing a color change in the sample.
    - The color change of the sample indicates the amount of coagulation factor that has not reacted with ATIII. This correlates with the amount of ATIII in the sample.
    - The control sample is used to establish the color of a solution with 100% ATIII activity. On the basis of the color difference of the patient's sample compared to the control, the percentage of ATIII activity in the patient's sample is reported.
- M. Thromboelastography (TEG)
  - Specialized analysis of the function of proteins and cellular components involved in hemostasis.
  - Whole blood is collected into a citrated tube (9 parts blood: 1 part 3.2% sodium citrate) to be analyzed at a set time point (often 30 minutes after collection).
  - The sample is added to a prewarmed (37°C) sample cup that contains calcium to initiate clot formation.
  - Analyzers for TEG typically have a detection probe that is placed into the blood sample to detect differences in the movement of the probe as the blood clots.
  - A schematic example of the data acquired from TEG is shown in Figure 3.6.
    - Typical data measurements include the time it takes to initiate clot formation (R), clotting time (K), the time to cross-link fibrin (α-angle), the maximum amplitude (MA) of the curve, and the amplitude of the curve 60 minutes after the MA was reached (A_{60}).
    - Different disease processes alter the values of these measurements in specific ways.
      - For example, a dog with a coagulation factor deficiency will likely have prolonged R and K values, a decreased MA, and a smaller α-angle than a healthy dog.

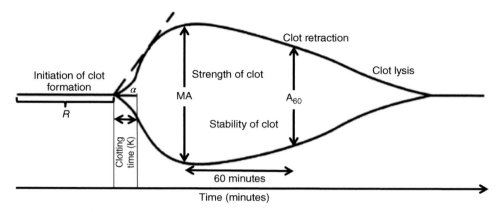

Figure 3.6   Thromboelastography tracing. The types of data that are collected by thromboelastography are indicated. Typical measurements taken include the time it takes to initiate clot formation (R), clotting time (K), the time to cross-link fibrin (α), the maximum amplitudeMA of the curve (MA), and the amplitude of the curve 60 minutes after the MA was reached (A_{60}).

TECHNICIAN TIP 3–2: ANTICOAGULANTS USED FOR HEMOSTASIS ASSAYS

- Different anticoagulants are preferred for different tests.
  - Purple-topped tubes contain EDTA.
    - Preferred for platelet counts.
    - The final concentration of EDTA should be 1.8 mg/mL of blood.
  - Green-topped tubes contain heparin.
    - Preferred if the same sample is needed for a plasma biochemistry profile.
    - The final concentration of heparin should be approximately 16 international units/mL of blood.
    - Heparin may cause platelet clumping.
  - Blue-topped tubes contain 3.2% sodium citrate.
    - Preferred for most platelet function tests.
    - Tubes that contain citrate are designed to dilute a blood sample by 10%.
      - Be sure to take this dilution factor into account when platelet (counts are determined from citrated samples.
    - Citrate may alter mean platelet volume (MPV) and can cause platelet clumping in canine blood samples.

Further Reading

Bay J.D., Scott M.A. & Hans J.E. (2000) Reference values for activated coagulation time in cats. *American Journal of Veterinary Research*, 61(7):750–753.

Boudreaux, M.K. (2011) *Hemostasis: Lecture Notes 2011.* Linus Publications, Inc., Deer Park, NY.

Clauss, A. (1957) Rapid physiological coagulation method in determination of fibrinogen. *Acta Haematologica*, 17 (4), 237–246.

Furlanello T., Caldin M., Stocco A., *et al.* (2006) Stability of stored canine plasma for hemostasis testing. *Veterinary Clinical Pathology*, 35(2):204–207.

Gerber B., Taboada J., Lothrop C.D. Jr.,, *et al.* (1999). Determination of normal values using an automated coagulation timer for activated coagulation time and its application in dogs with hemophilia. *Journal of Veterinary Internal Medicine*, 13(5):433–436.

Harvey, J.W. (ed) (2012) *Veterinary Hematology: A Diagnostic Guide and Color Atlas.* Elsevier Saunders, St. Louis, MO.

Jergens A.E., Turrentine M.A., Kraus K.H. & Johnson G.S. (1987) Buccal mucosa bleeding times of healthy dogs and of dogs in various pathologic states, including thrombocytopenia, uremia, and von Willebrand's disease. *American Journal of Veterinary Research*, 48(9):1337–1342.

Millar H.R., Simpson J.G., Stalker A.L. (1971) An evaluation of the heat precipitation method for plasma fibrinogen estimation. *Journal of Clinical Pathology*, 24(9):827–830.

Nurden A.T. & Caen J.P. (1975) Specific roles for surface membrane glycoproteins in platelet function. *Nature*, 255:720–722.

Parker M.T., Collier L.L., Kier A.B. & Johnson G.S. (1988). Oral mucosa bleeding times of normal cats and cats with Chediak-Higashi syndrome or Hageman trait (Factor XII deficiency). *Veterinary Clinical Pathology*, 17(1):9–12.

Rooney M.M., Farrell D.H., van Hemel B.M., de Groot P.G. & Lord S.T. (1998). The contribution of the three hypothesized integrin-binding sites in fibrinogen to platelet-mediated clot retraction. *Blood*, 92(7):2374–2381.

Sato I., Anderson G.A. & Parry B.W. (2000). An interobserver and intraobserver study of BMBT in Greyhounds. *Research in Veterinary Science*, 68(1):41–45.

Weiss D.J. & Wardrop K.J. (eds) (2010) *Schalm's Veterinary Hematology* (6th ed.). Ames, IA: Wiley-Blackwell.

Interpretation and comments for Case 1

Interpretation: As discussed in Case 1 from Chapter 2, this patient has a macrocytic, hypochromic, regenerative anemia that is likely due to immune-mediated hemolysis. The leukon indicates inflammation and stress. The thrombocytopenia is a major concern and coagulation testing was pursued. PT and PTT are prolonged indicating dysfunction of extrinsic, intrinsic, and common coagulation pathways. FDPs are increased raising concern for increased fibrinolysis. The combination of thrombocytopenia, increased PT, increased PTT, and increased FDPs raises grave concern for DIC.

Comments: This patient is likely in a critical condition that requires immediate medical intervention.

Interpretation and comments for Case 2

Interpretation: The results indicate that the patient has a diseases affecting the extrinsic, intrinsic, and common coagulation pathways.

Comment: The owners indicated that they recently placed rat poison in the garage. Coumarin toxicity was determined to be the cause of the coagulopathy in this cat.

Interpretation and comments for Case 3

Interpretation: Given the signalment and results of the BMBT, vWD was suspected.

Comment: Before performing spay, the veterinarian ordered a crossmatch to ensure that compatible blood was available for transfusion if needed.

Activities

Multiple Choice Questions

1. Which type of blood collection tube should be used for PT and PTT assays?
   A) Blue-topped tube containing sodium citrate
   B) Green-topped tube containing heparin
   C) Purple-topped tube containing EDTA
   D) Red-topped tube containing no anticoagulant

2. The most common clinical sign associated with thrombocytopenia is development of:
   A) Aural hematomas
   B) Bilateral epistaxis
   C) Internal hemorrhage
   D) Subcutaneous ecchymoses

3. True or False. Coagulation abnormalities can lead to extensive hemorrhaging.

4. Ingestion of which of the following pesticides could prolong a patient's PT and PTT?
   A) Avermectin-based anthelminthic
   B) Coumarin-based rodenticide
   C) Pyrethrin-based insecticide
   D) Triazine-based herbicide

5. Which of the following facts about anticoagulants is true?
   A) Heparin may cause platelet clumping.
   B) EDTA should not be used to determine a platelet count.
   C) No anticoagulant should be used for coagulation testing.
   D) Tubes that contain citrate do not dilute the blood sample.

Clinical Chemistry

University of Illinois, Champaign, IL, USA

Learning Objectives

The student will be able to
1. Prepare a sample for chemistry analysis.
2. Understand the impact of lipemia and hemolysis on analytes of a chemistry profile.
3. Understand the impact of dehydration on the results of the chemistry profile.
4. Recognize which analytes are used to evaluate different organ systems.
5. Identify abnormal values and understand their clinical significance.
6. Appreciate the significance of the signalment of the patient when interpreting results.

KEY TERMS

Analyte
Electrolyte
Enzyme
Hemolytic index
Icteric index
Lipemic index
Kidney
Liver
Plasma
Protein
Renal
Serum

Clinical Pathology and Laboratory Techniques for Veterinary Technicians, First Edition.
Edited by Anne Barger and Amy MacNeill.
© 2015 John Wiley & Sons, Inc. Published 2015 by John Wiley & Sons, Inc.
Companion Website: www.wiley.com/go/barger/vettechclinpath

Case example 1

The patient pictured below is a 4-year-old, spayed female, Miniature Dachshund with a history of lethargy. Physical examination revealed marked icterus. What analyte measured in the blood is increased with clinical icterus?

Answer: Total bilirubin.

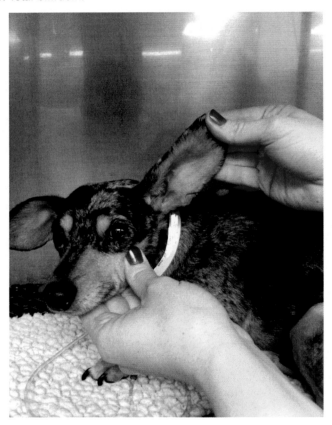

Case example 2

A 7-year-old domestic short cat presents for drinking increased amounts of water and urinating outside of the litter box. The patient has an elevated creatinine of 2.2 mg/dL (ref range: 0.4–0.9 mg/dL) and an elevated urea of 65 mg/dL (ref range: 7–28 mg/dL) with a USG of 1.023. What organ system is most likely affected and what is the term used to describe the elevated urea and creatinine?

Answer: Kidney and azotemia.

Introduction

Clinical biochemistry or a chemistry profile is an important component of a patient's minimum database. A minimum database generally refers to a combination of laboratory tests which allows the veterinarian to begin to evaluate the patient's overall organ function. The laboratory tests usually include a CBC, chemistry profile, and urinalysis. A general chemistry profile is often used as a primary diagnostic tool and includes *analytes* that evaluate *liver*, *kidney*, fluid balance, *electrolytes*, *proteins*, and acid–base status. Chemistry profiles can also be focused for evaluation of a single organ such as kidney or liver. These are usually performed on patients that already have a diagnosis and the profile is used to monitor response to therapy rather than make a primary diagnosis. A chemistry profile can be performed on serum, plasma, or whole blood depending on the type of analyzer being used.

Available Testing

A full chemistry profile can be performed in an in-house laboratory or sent out to a diagnostic laboratory. The in-house equipment available is always changing and often improving. Abaxis, Heska, and IDEXX all have veterinary chemistry testing equipment on the market. These analyzers require only a small amount of blood. Analyzers vary in the type of sample needed to perform testing. Many of the analyzers utilize cartridges that are already set up with a panel of tests; however, some allow for individual analytes to be analyzed. The manufacturer's instructions are essential for appropriately operating the instrumentation. Outside laboratories are also available. It is essential that personnel in these laboratories are appropriately trained in veterinary clinical pathology. The majority of chemistry analyzers in major laboratories use serum in dogs and cats and plasma for large animals such as horses and cattle. The blood of horses and cattle can take a long time to clot so running the samples on plasma is more efficient.

Sample Preparation

Blood should be drawn from the patient and placed in the appropriate tube for the sample type. A clean stick is essential to avoid hemolysis. The type of tube used depends on the type of sample required, serum or plasma. If serum is required, the sample will need to clot first. This will take 2–5 minutes but may be delayed if the patient has a hemostatic disorder. If plasma is desired, the sample can be centrifuged immediately.

A. Tubes
  - Serum
    - Serum separator tubes
      - As the sample is centrifuged, a special gel moves between the clot and the serum. The tube has a red and gray top (Figure 4.1).

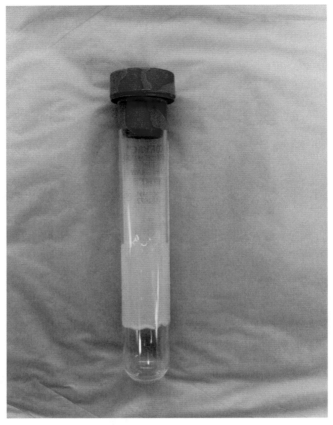

Figure 4.1   The serum separator tubes have a red and gray top, often called a "tiger top" with a white gel used to separate serum from blood cells with centrifugation.

- Serum separators should not be used for samples drawn to measure drug levels such as phenobarbital because the sample can be falsely decreased from contact with the serum separator.
- Red top tubes (Figure 4.2).
  - These tubes contain no anticoagulant and no serum separator. The sample needs to be centrifuged and the serum immediately removed from the clot (Table 4.1).
- Plasma
  - Heparin tubes (Figure 4.2)
    - These tubes have a green top and contain heparin to prevent the sample from clotting.
    - The sample can be centrifuged immediately and the plasma removed from the red blood cells with a pipette and placed in another tube for in-house testing and immediate analysis.

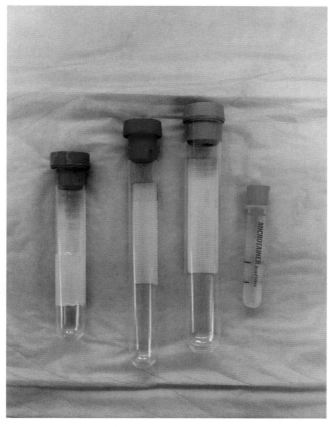

Figure 4.2   Blood tubes used for clinical chemistry testing from left to right are serum separator tube, red top tube used for serum, a large heparin tube with a green top containing the anticoagulant heparin, used to obtain plasma, and a micro-heparin tube used for small volumes of blood.

- When submitting heparinized samples to an outside laboratory, label the sample as heparinized plasma so the laboratory knows what they are dealing with.
- Filling of tubes
  - Avoid positive pressure when filling tubes, forcing the blood into the tube by pressing on the syringe can result in hemolysis. Let the tube fill via vacuum pressure or remove the rubber stopper on the tube (Figure 4.3a and b).

TECHNICIAN TIP 4–1   There are different types of heparin, sodium heparin and lithium heparin. For diagnostic testing, use lithium heparin because the sodium in the sodium heparin will interfere with the sodium measurement in the patient's plasma.

Table 4.1   Advantages and disadvantages of blood tubes for biochemical analysis.

	Advantages	Disadvantages
Serum tube (red top)	No interfering substances, easy to use	After centrifugation, the serum must be removed from the cells; otherwise, the cells will continue to metabolize glucose and may leach potassium into the serum
Serum separator (red and gray top)	After centrifugation, the sample can remain in the tube because the serum is automatically separated from the cells	These tubes cannot be used for hormone or drug analysis because the hormone/drug may diffuse from the serum into the gel resulting in a falsely lower value
Heparin (green top)	Do not have to wait for the sample to clot to centrifuge the sample	Use of sodium heparin tubes can interfere with accurate sodium measurements, not all tests validated for plasma

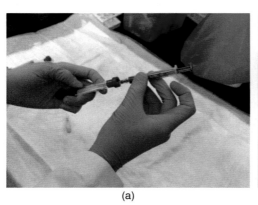 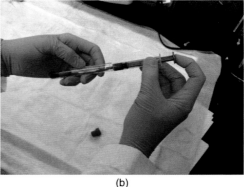

(a)   (b)

Figure 4.3   (a) The needle is inserted through the red stopper and vacuum pressure evacuates the blood. There is no need to put pressure on the plunger of the syringe. (b) Blood is injected in the tube by removing the red stopper from the tube and the needle from the syringe and depressing the plunger.

B. Centrifugation
- The sample should be centrifuged for 10 minutes at 3500rpm for both serum and plasma.
- Balance the centrifuge with a similar tube filled with a similar volume of fluid to the sample (Figure 4.4).
- After centrifugation, the sample should be removed from the red blood cells immediately, unless a serum separator is in place. In that case, the sample should be examined to insure complete separation of serum from cells by the gel.

C. Sample submission
- The sample should be refrigerated or frozen until sent to the laboratory.
- Send the sample with ice packs, with a courier or in the mail.
- Extreme heat will result in erroneous values.

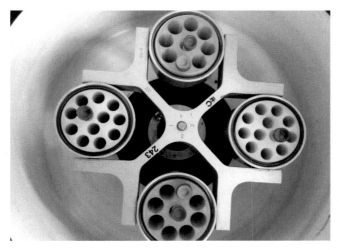

Figure 4.4   The centrifuge should be balanced with similar tubes filled with a similar volume of liquid to match the volume of blood.

Sample Quality

A. Venipuncture
  - A "clean stick" is important, redirected guidance of the needle or inserting the same needle through the skin multiple times can lead to a dull needle and traumatic venipuncture and hemolysis.
  - Blood can be drawn into a syringe, and the size of the syringe used will vary with the volume of blood needed. For a full chemistry profile performed on serum or plasma, 2–3 mL of blood should be enough for full analysis. The blood needs to be quickly transferred from the syringe to the appropriate tubes. If placing blood in an EDTA tube before the serum tube, be careful not to contaminate the needle with EDTA.
    - EDTA contamination will result in decreased calcium (values can drop as low as 1 or 2 mg/dL) and if it is potassium EDTA, it may result in an elevated potassium as well.
  - It is very important to determine what type of sample is required for the test/analyzer being used (plasma vs serum).
    - Heparinized plasma can be used for many diagnostic tests.
    - If serum is used, refer the section titled "Sample Preparation."
B. All chemistry tests have a range for which measurement of the test is accurate, this is referred to as a linear range. If an animal is sick, a particular analyte may be so high it exceeds the linear range. A dilution must be performed to return the analyte to a measurable range. Some of the larger analyzers, usually those used in commercial laboratories, will perform dilutions automatically, as soon as the range is exceeded however most in-house analyzers do not do this but merely flag the result in some way to indicate that it may be inaccurate.

- An aliquot of the sample should be diluted with 0.9% saline. Start with equal parts of sample and saline (a 1:2 dilution). If the analyte is still out of range, greater dilutions can be performed. The result should be multiplied by the dilution used. If a 1:10 dilution is performed, multiply the result of the analyte concentration in the diluted sample by 10.

C. Gross evaluation of the serum or plasma
   - After centrifugation, the color and turbidity of serum or plasma can be evaluated. The normal color in dogs and cats is a pale yellow and the consistency should be clear. In horses and ruminants, the serum or plasma is yellow owing to the higher levels of bilirubin in horses and diet of ruminants.
   - The identification of hemolysis, lipemia, and icterus should be noted before chemical evaluation.
   - Many chemistry analyzers rely on absorbance of light or absorbance spectrophotometry to obtain a result; therefore, the presence of substances that affect the color or turbidity of serum or plasma can have great impact on particular analytes.
   - Hemolysis
      - Lysis of red blood cells results in release of hemoglobin in the serum. Damage of enough red blood cells can discolor the serum or plasma red (in Figure 4.5, all tubes show varying amounts of hemolysis). Visual evidence of hemolysis occurs at 20 mg/dL. Severe hemolysis can interfere with several laboratory tests.
      - Hemolysis can occur in vivo (in the patient) in which case it is associated with anemia and also hemoglobinuria or it can occur in vitro (outside of the patient), during venipuncture or as a result of sample handling.

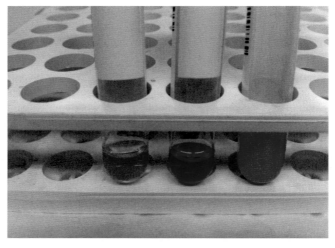

Figure 4.5   Serum samples with varying degrees of hemolysis. A. mild hemolysis, B. severe hemolysis, and C. hemolysis and lipemia.

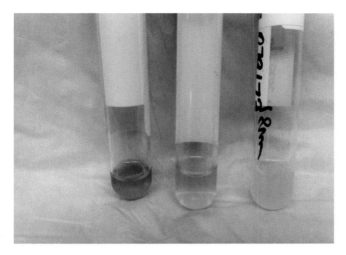

Figure 4.6   Serum from dogs exhibiting A. Hemolysis, B. Icterus, and C. Lipemia.

- The effect of hemoglobin on a particular analyte can be determined by adding known amounts of hemoglobin to a sample to determine which tests are impacted and at what level. Hemolysis is reported by most analyzers as 1+, 2+, 3+, and so on.
- Horses and some breeds of dogs, such as Akitas, have higher levels of potassium within erythrocytes so hemolysis can result in an elevation in potassium.
- Lipemia
  - Lipemia is the presence of excess lipid or fat in the blood. The serum or plasma appears opaque and is markedly turbid after centrifugation, giving the serum a "milky" appearance (Figure 4.6).
  - Lipemia can occur after a meal or postprandial and with different medical conditions including hyperlipoproteinemia of Schnauzers, familial hyperlipoproteinemia of Beagles, and secondary to several diseases including diabetes mellitus, hepatic lipidosis, and hypothyroidism.
  - Ideally, patients should be fasted before obtaining blood for analysis; however clinically, this is not always possible.
  - Lipemic samples can be refrigerated for 12–24 hours, the lipid component will rise to the top and the serum can be aspirated below the lipemic layer. Alternatively, an ultracentrifuge may be used to clear the lipemia. Most practices do not have this type of centrifuge; however, if outside laboratories are used, often they will use this piece of equipment to clear lipemia.
- Icterus
  - The description of icterus indicates a deep yellow color in response to elevated bilirubin. The serum color should correspond with an icteric index on the chemistry profile (Figure 4.6, middle tube).

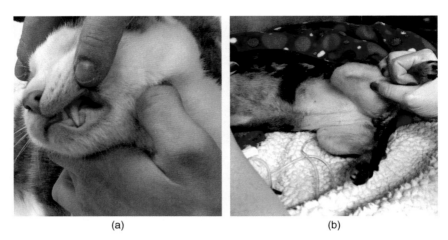

Figure 4.7   (a) A 7-year-old, female domestic shorthair cat, exhibiting marked icterus. Note the yellow coloring of the mucous membranes. (b) A 4-year-old Miniature Dachshund exhibiting marked clinical icterus. Icterus is easiest to recognize on nonhaired skin, mucous membranes, and sclera.

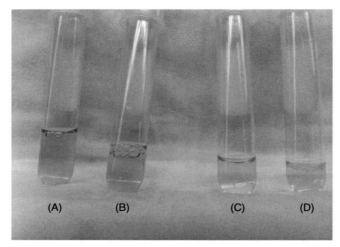

Figure 4.8   Serum from A. Cow, B. Horse, C. Cat, and D. Dog. Horses and cattle have similar deep yellow serum or plasma and dogs and cats normally have a pale yellow serum or plasma.

- The patient should also have an elevated bilirubin. If the bilirubin is elevated but the icteric index is not increased and/or the patient is not showing clinical evidence of icterus (Figure 4.7a and b), an incorrect elevation of the bilirubin should be considered such as lipemia or another interfering substance.
- Ruminants and horses may have an increased icteric indicator because of the color of the serum rather than the bilirubin content (Figure 4.8). This is normal for these animals.

Clinical Chemistry Health Profiles

A. Purpose
  - The function of these profiles is to evaluate overall organ function. These can be performed to establish the health of a patient before performing invasive procedures such as surgery, evaluate the optimal function of an organ system, diagnose a disease process, monitor the progression of an already diagnosed disease, or evaluate response to drug therapy known to be damaging to organs such as liver or kidney.
B. Compilation of tests
  - Generally, multiple analytes are used, rather than just one particular test.
    - One analyte provides very little information by itself.
  - Several analytes, combined in a panel, are used to evaluate one or multiple organ systems.
    - Renal profiles may include urea (BUN), creatinine (crt), albumin (alb), sodium (Na), potassium (K), chloride (Cl), phosphorus (P), and calcium (Ca).
    - Liver profiles may include alanine aminotransferase (ALT), alkaline phosphatase (ALP), total bilirubin (t. bili), urea, albumin, cholesterol, and glucose.
    - General health profiles include a combination of analytes used to evaluate liver, kidney, electrolytes, and proteins. A mixture of normal and abnormal results combined with clinical signs are used to diagnose a particular disease or lead the veterinarian to request more specific diagnostic tests.
C. Terminology
  - Results of chemistry analyses are compared to a species-specific reference range.
  - Values that are elevated are often termed "hyper," for example, an animal with an elevated phosphorus will be described as being hyperphosphatemic.
  - Values that are decreased are often preceded by "hypo," for example, a patient with a decreased albumin will be described as hypoalbuminemic.
  - These general rules do not apply uniformly to all analytes but will apply to most.
  - The suffix –emia indicates the presence of an analyte in the peripheral blood. For instance, hypoalbuminemia means that the patient has decreased circulating levels of albumin within the blood.

Blood Proteins

Definition: Proteins are chains of amino acids joined by peptide bonds in a linear sequence specified by DNA.

A. Polypeptide chains of amino acids
  - Over 1,000 different proteins are found in plasma.
  - May be combined with another substance such as a fat or sugar and described as a lipoprotein or glycoprotein, respectively.
B. Most proteins are produced in the liver, the exception is immunoglobulins (antibodies) that are produced by plasma cells in the lymphoid tissue and bone marrow.

C. Serum versus plasma protein
  • Plasma is the liquid portion (noncellular) of unclotted blood.
    • Plasma proteins contain fibrinogen, factor V, and factor VII (see Chapter 3) in addition to all of the proteins contained in serum.
  • Serum is the liquid portion of clotted blood and can be obtained after centrifugation. The proteins described in this section will be referred to as serum proteins even though they can occur in both serum and plasma.
D. Serum protein functions
  • Nutrition
  • Contribution to oncotic pressure. Oncotic pressure is a form of osmotic pressure where proteins pull water into the vessel.
  • Maintenance of acid–base status
  • Immune modulation (antibodies are composed of protein)
E. Specific proteins
  • The chemistry profile provides a value for total protein and albumin
  • Albumin
    • Produced in the liver
    • The most osmotically active protein
    • Prevents loss of substances through the kidney
  • Globulins
    • Most of the proteins in peripheral blood with the exception of albumin are globulins.
    • The majority of globulins are involved with inflammation or the immune system in one form or another.
    • Categorized based on their size and where they travel on an electrophoretogram, a method to separate proteins based on their molecular weight (Figure 4.9).
      • α-globulins: α2-macroglobulin, haptoglobin, and ceruloplasmin (acute phase proteins).
      • β-globulins: fibrinogen, protein C, and C-reactive protein (acute phase proteins).
      • γ-globulins: immunoglobulins (antibodies).

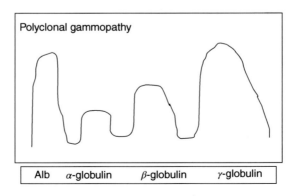

Figure 4.9   Electrophoretogram displaying peaks for alpha, beta, and gamma globulins.

F. Measurement of proteins
- Total plasma protein
  - Refractometry
    - Principle: degree of light refraction (refractive index) in a liquid is proportional to the amount of solids in the liquid.
    - Refractometers are available in most veterinary practices.
    - Method
      - Whole blood with anticoagulant is used for this procedure.
      - Fill two microhematocrit tubes $\frac{3}{4}$ full of blood, seal one end with clay.
      - Place the microhematocrit tubes opposite each other in the microhematocrit centrifuge with the clay facing outwards (Figure 4.10a).
      - Tighten the lid on the microhematocrit centrifuge, close the outside cover, and spin the samples for 5 minutes (Figure 10b).
      - Break the microhematocrit tube just slightly above the packed cells. With the portion of the tube containing the plasma, fill the refractometer with the liquid (Figure 4.10c and d).
      - Compress the plastic cover with your finger and angle the refractometer toward the light (Figure 4.10e).
      - Make sure that the refractometer is appropriately focused by adjusting the ocular.
      - Read the appropriate scale, the units for the total protein are in grams per deciliter (Figure 4.10f).
    - Because this technique relies on light to be able to pass through the liquid, both hemolysis and lipemia can interfere with accurate measurement of plasma total protein.
  - Serum total protein
    - Can be measured on most chemistry analyzers. The test is colorimetric and the range of measurement is 1–10 g/dL so values less than 1 g/dL cannot be detected and often a result of <1.0 g/dL will be reported.
- Albumin
  - Automated analyzers use the bromcresol green (BCG) binding assay. BCG binds to albumin and produces a color complex when bound. This color change is detected by the analyzer.
- Globulin
  - The value for globulins is determined via calculation.
  - Globulins = Total serum protein − albumin
- Fibrinogen
  - Fibrinogen is an acute phase protein that can be measured in plasma but not serum.
  - See Chapter 3 for the methodology.
- Albumin to globulin ratio (A:G)
  - This is a calculation, and the value obtained for the albumin is divided by the calculated globulin. The ratio should be around one. An increase or decrease may indicate a selective loss or elevation in either albumin or globulin rather than loss or increase in both analytes.

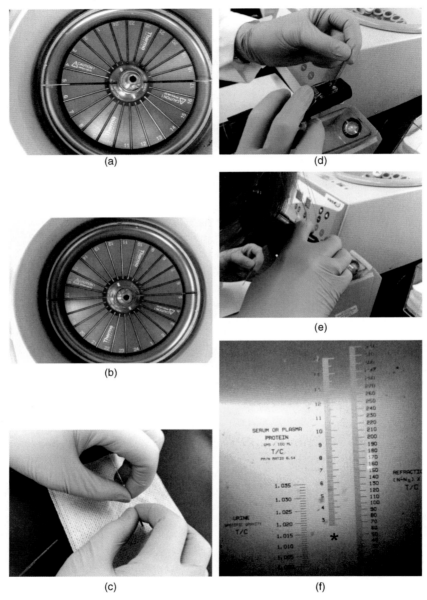

Figure 4.10 (a) Microhematocrit tubes filled with blood and sealed with clay, balanced in a microhematocrit centrifuge. The clay should be placed outwardly for centrifugation. (b) The same tubes after 5 minutes of centrifugation. The blood is divided into plasma, buffy coat, and packed red blood cells. (c) The tube is broken between the plasma and buffy coat, being careful not to contaminate the serum with cells from the buffy coat. Gloves should be worn for personal protection. (d) The refractometer is loaded using the plasma from the microhematocrit tube. Use the end of the tube that is not broken to avoid scratching the refractometer with small pieces of glass. (e) Angle the refractometer toward the light source. This may be attached to the refractometer as pictured or may require the user to take advantage of lighting in the room. (f) The refractometer scale indicated with an * is used for measuring the total protein.

G. Physiologic factors affecting the serum or plasma protein
  - Patient age
    - At birth, animals have a low protein due to minimal contribution of immunoglobulin. When neonates are born, the mother's first milk is referred to as colostrum. This milk is rich in immunoglobulin. After the neonate ingests colostrum, there is a significant increase in immunoglobulin in the peripheral blood.
    - Animals 6 months to a year of age usually reach adult levels of proteins.
    - Slight elevations can be seen postvaccination.
  - Reproductive status
    - Gestation and lactation: decreases in serum or plasma protein primarily due to decreased albumin.
H. Interpretation of abnormal values
  - Total protein
    - Either plasma or serum (remember plasma protein contains fibrinogen and other coagulation factors, serum protein does not).
    - Hypoproteinemia indicates a decrease in the total protein value. Causes can include loss or decreased production.
      - Loss of protein
        - Bleeding: usually external hemorrhage, resulting in a decrease in both albumin and globulin. The A:G will be close to 1.
        - Protein losing enteropathy is a severe inflammatory disease of the intestines that results in loss of both albumin and globulin together, again the A:G will be close to 1.
        - Protein losing nephropathy describes a loss of protein via the kidney. This can result from damage to the glomeruli or the renal tubules. Generally, the hypoproteinemia is from a loss of albumin, and globulins are often normal; therefore, the A:G will be significantly <1.
      - Decreased production
        - Albumin is produced primarily in the liver; therefore, animals with *severe* liver disease (>80% of the liver is damaged) can result in marked hypoalbuminemia. The globulins remain normal so the A:G is decreased.
      - Failure of passive transfer. If foals or calves fail to nurse, they will not receive the vitally important immunoglobulins from the dam's milk. This early milk, rich in immunoglobulins, is called colostrum. As a result of this, young animals will have a hypoglobulinemia and be at risk for infection.
  - Hypoalbuminemia
    - Loss
      - Pure albumin loss is primarily renal in origin (protein-losing nephropathy).
      - Low albumin can also be seen in conjunction with low globulin. This is referred to as a panhypoproteinemia indicating that all proteins are decreased. Loss of protein-rich fluid can occur into the abdomen, pleural cavity, or pericardial space. These locations are often referred to as "third space."
    - Decreased production due to decreased liver function. Globulins are typically normal in these patients. Even though many globulins are produced in the

liver, the primary globulins are immunoglobulins that are produced by plasma cells as part of the immune response.
- Hypoglobulinemia
  - Loss of globulins often occurs concurrently with loss of albumin so hemorrhage, third space loss, and protein losing enteropathy are likely causes. The A:G is close to one when both albumin and globulin are lost together.
  - Decreased production is usually associated with immunocompromised animals, such as a foal with failure of passive transfer or an inherited immunodeficiency.
- Hyperproteinemia
  - The most common cause of hyperproteinemia is relative, secondary to dehydration. A dehydrated patient has less fluid in its blood; therefore, the solid component appears relatively increased.
  - Dehydration can result in hyperalbuminemia and hyperglobulinemia.
- Hyperglobulinemia
  - An elevated globulin with a normal or decreased albumin is often associated with immune stimulation and/or antigenic stimulation.
    - Elevated immunoglobulins and/or acute phase proteins.
  - Neoplastic production of immunoglobulins can also be seen with a plasma cell neoplasia (called multiple myeloma) or lymphoma.
- Fibrinogen
  - Fibrinogen is an acute phase protein so it is expected to increase greatly as part of an inflammatory response.
  - Elevations can be the result of inflammation or dehydration. Fibrinogen is used more commonly in horses and ruminants to evaluate for inflammation. Changes in acute phase proteins, such as fibrinogen, are more sensitive than changes to the CBC in these species.

Kidney

A. Basic physiology
  - The kidney has multiple functions but its prime objective is the elimination of waste by the production of urine. A full urinalysis, in combination with specific analytes in the chemistry profile to evaluate renal function, is essential for accurate diagnosis.
  - Nephron
    - The nephron is the functional unit of the kidney and it is composed of the glomerulus and tubules. The purpose of these structures is filtering the blood, excreting waste products such as urea and creatinine, balancing water loss or conservation based on the hydration status of the patient, and conservation of specific electrolytes and proteins.
    - Refer to the Chapter 5 for more specific information on the function of individual components of the nephron and its role in urine production.
    - The kidney is an amazing organ. It can function normally if >34% of the nephrons are working efficiently.

B. Evaluation of renal function
- Definitions of disease
  - Renal Disease: The presence of morphological renal lesions of any size or severity or any biochemical abnormalities indicative of abnormal renal function. Pathology that occurs within the kidney is often described as a nephropathy. "Nephro" refers to the nephron and "pathy" indicates disease or pathology.
  - Renal Failure: clinical signs and/or biochemical abnormalities are indicative of decreased renal function.
    - The nephron is described as the functional unit of the kidney. Therefore, a decrease in renal function indicates a decreased number of functioning nephrons.
    - Acute renal failure happens very quickly and is often sustained. The renal parameters evaluated in the blood are often markedly elevated.
  - Specific renal insults that can result in failure
    - Toxic nephropathy: severe toxic insult to renal tubules as observed with such toxins as ethylene glycol (antifreeze) and aminoglycoside antibiotics.
    - Acute ischemic event: Ischemia is a lack of blood flow to a tissue resulting in the death of the cells of that tissue. Damage associated with a lack of blood flow happens very quickly and therefore can result in acute renal failure. Ischemia within the kidney can occur from shock, decreased cardiac output, transfusion reaction, a blood clot, and so on.
    - Chronic renal failure: primary renal failure that has persisted for a long period of time, often months or years.
      - The patient's history and physical presentation are important in differentiating chronic and acute renal failure.
  - Azotemia: Excess urea or other nonprotein nitrogenous compounds (e.g., creatinine) in the blood.
    - Azotemia is characterized as prerenal, renal, or postrenal.
  - Glomerular filtration rate: or GFR is a unit of measure to describe how quickly blood is being filtered through the glomerulus each minute. It is used as a method to evaluate renal health and function. Analytes such as creatinine can be used to evaluate the GFR.
- Laboratory tests used to evaluate renal function.
  - Urea or blood urea nitrogen (BUN) is a nitrogenous waste product excreted by the kidney. Urea is produced in the liver and is a waste product of protein metabolism. Protein is absorbed by the intestine and ammonia is a waste product of protein metabolism. Ammonia is toxic to mammals, and therefore, the ammonia must be converted into a nontoxic waste product that can be safely excreted from the body. The liver converts ammonia into urea with the urea cycle.
    - Excretion of urea is primarily by the kidney but minimally in saliva and in the gastrointestinal (GI) tract of horses.
    - Laboratory methods
      - Serum chemistry is a common method used to detect urea concentration.

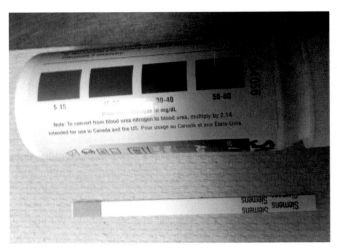

Figure 4.11   The blood is placed on the pad on the test strip and a color change is compared to the chart on the vial and the appropriate number recorded.

- Azostix are a reagent strip impregnated with urease bromothyomol blue and coated with a membrane that is permeable to urea but not blood. The result is a range rather than an individual number (Figure 4.11).
- Processes that increase urea concentration.
  - Prerenal azotemia
    - The elevation in urea happens before blood being filtered by the kidney.
      - Dehydration (urine should be concentrated) is a common cause of elevated urea. During dehydration, the patient has a decreased GFR due to an overall decrease in blood volume.
      - Increased protein metabolism will result in increased amounts of ammonia being converted by the liver into urea. Examples of this include a high protein diet, GI hemorrhage with possible ulceration, and increased protein catabolism associated with fever or prolonged infection.
  - Renal azotemia occurs as a result of severe kidney disease.
    - 75% of nephrons are nonfunctional or damaged before an increase in urea is observed; therefore, azotemia is not a very sensitive indicator of renal disease.
    - A loss of concentrating ability by the nephrons (inability to appropriately concentrate the urine) will precede azotemia and will occur when >66% of the nephrons are damaged.
    - Ruminants do not have as drastic an increase in urea compared to nonruminants because the rumen has the ability to recycle urea and use it as a protein source.
  - Postrenal azotemia
    - This occurs when there is an obstruction of urine flow (e.g., blocked cat) or leaking urine into the abdomen (uroabdomen or uroperitoneum)

- Uroabdomen results in a reabsorption of everything that was in the urine being reabsorbed by the abdomen into the blood.
- Processes that will result in a decreased urea usually result from decreased production or increased excretion.
  - Decreased production of urea by the liver can result in a severe decrease in urea. The liver converts toxic ammonia into safe and excretable urea. If the liver is severely compromised, the urea production will decrease and serum ammonia concentration will increase.
  - Low protein diet
    - Protein absorbed by the GI tract results in increased production of ammonia, which is then converted into urea. Animals that have a low protein diet will have minimal ammonia to convert into urea. Therefore, the overall blood urea level will be lower than an animal with a high protein diet.
  - Increased excretion
    - If a decreased GFR results in an increased urea, it only makes sense that an increased GFR would result in a decreased urea.
    - Patients that develop polyuria and polydipsia (PU/PD), or increased urination and drinking, and have a functional kidney, will excrete a higher amount of urea than a healthy patient. Many diseases are associated with PU/PD, some include diabetes mellitus, hyperadrenocorticism, and diabetes insipidus.
    - Patients receiving fluid therapy may also have a decreased urea.
- Creatinine
  - General information
    - Creatinine is a nonprotein source of nitrogen.
    - It is a product of creatine metabolism used during muscle contraction and is essentially a "waste product" of normal muscle metabolism. The amount produced is fairly constant in most animals.
  - Excretion
    - Excretion of creatinine is almost entirely via the kidney through the glomerular filtrate. A small amount is excreted by the renal tubules in male dogs (Table 4.2).
  - Measurement of creatinine

Table 4.2   Why is creatinine better than urea when measuring GFR?

- It takes longer for creatinine to equilibrate: urea is freely filtered and will be reabsorbed quickly

- The renal tubules minimally reabsorb creatinine but will reabsorb urea

- Creatinine is not as significantly impacted by the diet and urea can increase with a high protein meal

- Serum or plasma chemistry is the primary method of measurement. It is a colorimetric test that has minimal interference from other substances, referred to as noncreatinine chromagens.
- Elevations in creatinine are characterized similarly to elevations in urea.
  - Prerenal azotemia
    - A dehydrated patient will often have an elevated creatinine due to decreased GFR.
    - Severe damage of muscles (rhabdomyolysis) can result in mild elevation in creatinine, although it is usually a mild or insignificant elevation.
  - Renal azotemia
    - Similar to urea, elevations in creatinine are considered azotemia so patients with renal failure are expected to have clinically significant elevations in creatinine.
    - Similar sensitivity to urea (>75% of nephrons damaged before azotemia observed).
    - Elevations in creatinine are considered more sensitive in ruminants than urea because urea can be recycled by the rumen and creatinine is not recycled.
    - It is very important to correlate elevated creatinine with urine-specific gravity (USG) to differentiate renal azotemia from prerenal azotemia (refer to Chapter 5).
  - Postrenal azotemia
    - Same as for urea.
    - Excellent diagnostic tool for uroabdomen because creatinine is not as quickly reabsorbed from the abdomen as urea. Urea is freely filtered. The creatinine levels in the abdominal fluid should be compared to serum creatinine. In a patient with uroperitoneum or ruptured bladder, the creatinine levels in the abdominal fluid will be higher than the serum levels.

TECHNICIAN TIP 4–2 In patients suspected of uroabdomen, creatinine levels should be measured in the abdominal fluid and compared to the serum. Patients with uroabdomen will have greater levels of creatinine in the abdomen compared with the serum. This disease is most commonly diagnosed in foals less than 1 week of age.

- Decreased creatinine
  - This is an uncommon finding but can be observed with in animals with severe muscle wasting and may actually mask an underlying renal azotemia.
  - Similar to urea, patient's receiving aggressive fluid therapy or with severe PU/PD can have a mildly decreased creatinine.
- Interpretation of USG with azotemia
  - Patients with prerenal azotemia should be able to concentrate their urine. A clinically dehydrated patient should have an increased USG. USG

values in dogs <1.025 and in cats <1.035 are usually considered poorly concentrated and may suggest an underlying renal issue.
- Animals >3% dehydrated produce a hormone, anti-diuretic hormone or ADH that will influence the renal tubules to resorb water and concentrate the urine.
- Patients in renal failure are unable to appropriately concentrate their urine and are commonly described as having isosthenuria (specific gravity 1.008–1.012) in the face of azotemia. Refer to Chapter 5 for more information on USG.
- Other serum chemical abnormalities associated with renal disease
  - Phosphorus
    - Elevated phosphorus (hyperphosphatemia) is common because phosphorus is primarily excreted by the kidney in dogs and cats. Phosphorus can be elevated in animals with prerenal or renal azotemia.
    - Azotemic horses and cattle can have normal phosphorus because the kidney is not the primary source of excretion.
  - Potassium
    - Potassium can increase in patients with decreased urine production.
    - Animals with increased urine production (polyuria) will often have decreased potassium (hypokalemia).
  - Calcium
    - Hypocalcemia can occur in dogs, cats, and ruminants with chronic renal failure.
    - Hypercalcemia can occur in horses with renal failure but is less common in dogs and cats.
  - Albumin
    - Kidneys filter protein and prevent its loss in the urine. Severe glomerular and tubular disease can result in significant protein loss via the kidney. Glomerular disease is more likely to result a severe decrease in albumin in the peripheral blood.
  - Anemia (see Chapter 2)
    - The kidney is the source of erythropoietin which is a hormone responsible for signaling the bone marrow to produce more red blood cells.
    - Patients with chronic kidney disease will often develop a mild-to-moderate anemia because they do not have enough erythropoietin, for this reason, the anemia is nonregenerative and the patient will not have a reticulocytosis.

Liver

The liver is a multilobulated organ located in the cranial abdomen. The liver is composed multiple cell types but is predominated by epithelial cells called hepatocytes. These cells are responsible for the majority of liver functions. It is an organ with multiple functions and vital to survival. The liver can be affected by disease in many different ways. Some analytes allow us to determine specific injuries to hepatocytes while others allow for detection of declining liver function.

A. Functions of the liver
- Digestion
  - The liver produces bile which is essential in the digestion of fat. Bile is delivered from the liver to the intestine from bile ducts in the liver, to the gall bladder, and then to the duodenum through the common bile duct.
- Metabolism of many different substances
  - Carbohydrate metabolism
    - Storage of glycogen and production of glucose
  - Protein metabolism and production is a vital role of the liver.
    - Albumin and many globulins (α- and β-globulins)
    - All coagulation factors except calcium
    - Formation of urea from ammonia produced as a product of protein metabolism.
  - Fat metabolism
    - Synthesis of cholesterol
    - Synthesis of fat from protein and carbohydrates
- Storage
  - Vitamins
  - Iron
- Detoxification and excretion of many different substances
  - Detoxification of endogenous and exogenous substances for excretion in bile.
  - Bilirubin is formed by the breakdown of heme from the natural turnover of red blood cells. The liver conjugates bilirubin so it can be removed by the kidneys.

B. Diagnostic testing of liver disease
- Detection of increased enzyme activity
  - Hepatocytes (primary epithelial cells in the liver) and biliary epithelial cells contain enzymes within their cytoplasm and on the surface of their cytoplasm (Figure 4.12). If the hepatocytes are damaged, the enzyme levels will increase in the blood.
  - Location of the enzyme within the cytoplasm or on the membrane of the cells is important to characterize the type of injury to the hepatocytes. Therefore, like with most organ systems, a panel of analytes, including enzymes and products of the liver, are used to fully evaluate the liver.
- Cytosolic enzymes
  - Enzymes located within the cytoplasm of the hepatocytes are referred to as cytosolic. Elevation of these enzymes indicates damage to or leakage from the hepatocytes.
  - Alanine aminotransferase (ALT)
    - This enzyme is used primarily in dogs and cats to evaluate hepatocellular damage.
    - ALT is fairly liver specific in dogs and cats although elevations with muscle damage have been reported in dogs.
    - ALT is not useful in ruminants and horses because the enzyme is not very liver specific in these species.

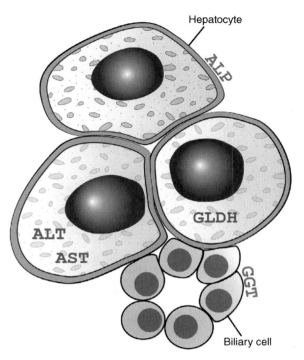

Figure 4.12   This drawing represents hepatocytes and biliary epithelial cells. The locations of the enzymes either cytosolic or membranous are demonstrated. ALT, AST, and SDH are cytosolic enzymes. ALP and GGT are membranous enzymes.

- ALT can increase with many different liver diseases but usually as a result of hepatocellular damage. Inflammation, toxic insults to the liver secondary to drug administration such as phenobarbital and certain anesthetics (sevoflurane, isoflurane, and halothane) have been reported to cause elevations.
  - Other diseases that can result in elevated ALT include hyperadrenocorticism, hyperthyroidism, and cardiac failure.
  - About 50% of cats with hyperthyroidism have a mild-to-moderate elevation in ALT.
- Aspartate aminotransferase (AST)
  - Another cytosolic enzyme found not only in liver but also in muscle. Significant elevations can be seen in patients with liver disease or significant muscle disease.
  - AST is also present in red blood cells so hemolysis can result in elevations in this enzyme.
  - AST is more specific in horses and cattle in the identification of liver damage, whereas ALT is a more specific enzyme to diagnose liver disease in small animals.
    - AST should be used in conjunction with other liver and muscle enzymes to determine whether the source is liver or muscle.

- Sorbitol dehydrogenase (SDH)
  - Liver specific enzyme for all species but used more commonly in horses and cattle.
  - Half-life is very short so this may limit the clinical utility of this enzyme. If the sample cannot be run immediately, it should be frozen. Most in-house analyzers do not offer this enzyme so usually it is sent out and therefore the serum/plasma should be frozen.
- Inducible enzymes are enzymes that are located on the cellular membrane rather than within the cytoplasm. Lysis of hepatocytes will not result in increases in these enzymes.
  - Alkaline phosphatase
    - This enzyme is membrane bound and its release into the serum is inducible by drugs and bile salts.
    - ALP is present in many tissues including liver, bone, kidney, intestine, and placenta. The kidney has the greatest quantity of ALP; however, ALP from the kidney is released in the urine rather than in the blood. Bone and liver ALP can be specifically identified in the serum of most species. Intestinal ALP contributes little to the serum total ALP. Within the liver, ALP is present on hepatocytes and biliary epithelial cells.
    - In dogs, a corticosteroid isoenzyme of alkaline phosphatase (CALP) can be identified in the serum. This enzyme can increase in dogs with endogenous elevations in cortisol, which can be seen in a stressed patient or a dog with hyperadrenocorticism. This isoenzyme will also increase in dogs being treated with glucocorticoids such as prednisolone. CALP is a component of the total ALP reported on the chemistry profile.
    - Elevations in ALP can accompany many diseases resulting in abnormal bile flow from the liver to the duodenum or cholestasis. Cholestatic diseases can be caused by physical obstruction of bile flow or by metabolic diseases of the liver such as hepatic lipidosis.
    - Certain breeds of dogs can have elevations in ALP as a normal finding, for example, Scottish terriers.
    - ALP is used minimally in ruminants because they have such a wide reference interval.
    - Young growing animals can have significant elevations in ALP and this is a normal finding due to bone growth.
    - Cats versus dogs
      - Cats have less liver ALP than dogs.
      - Cats do not have CALP.
      - The half-life of ALP in the cat is really short (6 hours) compared to the dog (72 hours), therefore, any elevation in ALP in the cat is significant (Table 4.3).
  - Gamma glutamyl transferase (GGT)
    - Also a membrane-bound enzyme.
    - Present on not only hepatocytes but also biliary epithelial cells.
    - Inducible, such as ALP, so will increase with glucocorticoid administration.

Table 4.3   An incomplete list of diseases resulting in elevations in total ALP.

Cholestatic diseases
Drug administration (especially glucocorticoids)
Diabetes mellitus
Hyperadrenocorticism (most common in dogs)
Pancreatitis
Hepatic lipidosis
Osteolytic lesions and/or young growing animals
Hyperthyroidism (cats)

- Will increase with cholestatic diseases and is considered a better indicator of cholestatic disease in horses and cattle than ALP.
- GGT, such as ALP, is also present in renal tubular epithelial cells. If the renal cells are damaged, GGT is released in the urine; therefore, detection of increased levels of urine GGT is indicative of renal tubular damage.
- Blood levels of GGT may be increased in neonates, primarily lambs, puppies, and calves. The dam's colostrum is rich in GGT so neonates that have ingested colostrum will have increases in this enzyme.
- Tests to evaluate hepatocellular function
  - As mentioned earlier in this section, the liver has many functions and products. On a standard chemistry profile, many liver products are measured.
  - Bilirubin
    - Bilirubin is derived from the heme portion of red blood cell hemoglobin.
    - Moderate elevations of bilirubin should result in a color change in the patient's skin, mucosa, and sclera but also the serum or plasma. A yellowing of the tissues (called icterus) is clinical support that a patient has an elevated bilirubin.
    - Types of bilirubin
      - Unconjugated bilirubin has not been fully processed by the liver. It is bound to albumin and therefore cannot be excreted by the kidney.
      - Conjugated bilirubin is conjugated by the hepatocytes so it can be excreted in bile. It is water soluble and filtered by the glomerulus of the kidney.
      - Delta bilirubin is conjugated bilirubin bound to albumin.
      - The combination of these three forms is commonly measured by most in-house analyzers as t. bili.
    - Elevation of bilirubin in the blood (hyperbilirubinemia), similar to azotemia, is classified as prehepatic, hepatic, or posthepatic based on where the site of disease is.
      - Prehepatic hyperbilirubinemia occurs because of excess hemoglobin breakdown secondary to hemolysis or internal hemorrhage.

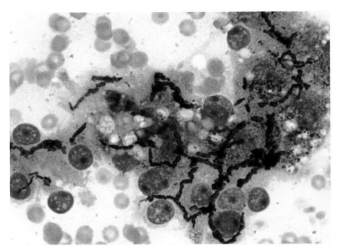

Figure 4.13   Cytology of a liver aspirate from a dog with pancreatitis. A cluster of hepatitis, surrounded by bile canaliculi filled with dark green bile pigment, demonstrate the cholestasis (Wright-Giemsa stain, 100×).

- Immune-mediated hemolytic anemia
- Blood transfusion reaction
- Red blood cell parasite or toxin
- Hepatic hyperbilirubinemia occurs in patients with decreased functional mass of liver or impaired hepatocytes that are unable to uptake and transport bilirubin.
  - Primary hepatic cholestasis
  - Anorexia in horses and cattle
  - Hepatic lipidosis in cats, ponies, and dogs
- Posthepatic hyperbilirubinemia occurs with an obstruction resulting in decreased excretion or transport of bilirubin (Figure 4.13).
  - Mechanical obstructions are most common and include cholelith, pancreatitis, and an unfortunately placed neoplasm.
- False elevations in bilirubin can occur with marked lipemia. These elevations will not result in clinical icterus or icteric serum.
- Bile acids (BAs)
- BAs are synthesized by the liver from cholesterol, secreted in bile, and stored in the gall bladder.
- When an animal eats, especially a meal that is high in fat, the chemical cholecystokinin is released, which results in gall bladder contraction and release of BA into the intestine via the bile duct.
- The majority of the BA are reabsorbed by the intestine (specifically the ileum) and returned to the liver by the portal vein and then recycled by the liver. The majority of the BA is removed from circulation on the first pass through the liver so BA levels in the blood return to normal very quickly after a meal.
- BA is not a component of the standard chemistry profile but rather a specific diagnostic test with specific steps that will greatly impact the results. Performing the test in dogs and cats:

- Serum is used for this test.
- The patient should be fasted for at least 8 hours. A preprandial BA sample is drawn and placed in a red top tube or serum separator tube. The tube should be labeled "preprandial BAs."
- The patient is then fed a fairly high fat meal.
- Two hours after the meal, a postprandial BA sample is drawn and placed in a red top or serum separator tube. The tube should be labeled "postprandial BAs."
- In a normal liver, the majority of the BAs should be removed from circulation in less than 2 hours. Some animals with liver disease will have a normal preprandial BAs but a markedly elevated postprandial BAs so it is essential to perform this test with paired samples.
- Increased BA
  - The reference range for a postprandial BA is often slightly higher than the preprandial BA.
  - Any time the t. bili. is increased from a hepatic or posthepatic cause, the BA will likely be elevated.
  - Abnormal blood flow to the liver from congenital or acquired lesions will result in elevations in BAs. Portosystemic shunts are abnormal blood vessels that take blood directly from the intestine to the rest of the body bypassing detoxification by the liver.
  - Decreased hepatic blood flow, for example, patients with right-sided heart failure.
- BAs in horses
  - Horses do not have a gall bladder so this will complicate this test. There is continuous circulation of BA, therefore, no need for pre- and postprandial BAs.
  - BAs are not specific for any one hepatic disease but if elevated, they are supportive of hepatic disease in horses.
  - Horses with hyperbilirubinemia from anorexia will have mild elevations in BA.
- BAs in ruminants
  - The rumen acts as a feed reservoir so there is a continuous flow of feed to the small intestine; therefore, it is really challenging to get a fasted sample in a ruminant.
  - In addition, there is a wide reference range in cattle with many variables that impact BA, particularly lactation status. Lactating cattle can have BA >100 µM/L.
- Pseudofunction tests (liver products)
  - Several products of the liver, measured in a typical chemistry profile, will be significantly decreased in patients with decreased functional hepatocellular mass resulting from congenital portosystemic shunts or severe liver disease, resulting in liver failure.
  - Albumin
    - The liver is the primary source of albumin production. >80% of the liver is nonfunctional before a measurable decrease in albumin is detectable.

- Urea
  - As protein is absorbed from the intestine, it is deaminated (amine groups are removed) in the liver, which results in production of ammonia. Ammonia is highly toxic and therefore the liver converts the ammonia into urea that can be safely excreted in the urine.
- Glucose
  - The liver is responsible for gluconeogenesis (production of glucose) and glycogenolysis. Patients with decreased functional hepatocellular mass have a severe hypoglycemia.
- Cholesterol
  - Lipoproteins are synthesized in the liver so patients with severe liver disease can have marked hypocholesterolemia.
  - A combined decrease in cholesterol, albumin, urea, and glucose is a strong indication of decreased functional hepatocellular mass.
- Other abnormal diagnostic tests potentially seen with liver disease
  - Decreased mean corpuscular volume (MCV)
    - The liver is a source of iron metabolism. In patients with severe liver disease or vascular anomalies such as portosystemic shunts, the MCV can be decreased, essentially mimicking an iron deficiency anemia.
  - Abnormal red blood cell morphology
    - Acanthocytes (Figure 4.14) and target cells can both be seen in patients with liver disease
  - Prolonged prothrombin time and partial thromboplastin time
    - Most coagulation factors are produced in the liver so animals with severe liver disease can have prolongation of these assays (refer to Chapter 3).
  - Elevated ammonia levels

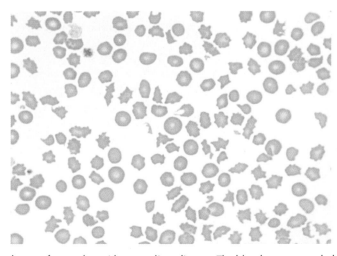

Figure 4.14   Blood smear from a dog with severe liver disease. The blood smear revealed marked acanthocytosis (Wright-Giemsa stain, 100×).

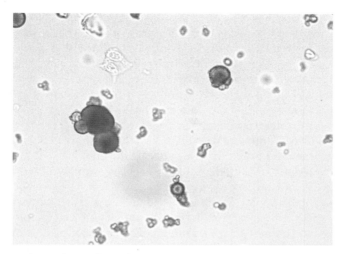

Figure 4.15   Urine sediment from a dog with a portosystemic shunt. Many ammonium biurate crystals were observed in this patient's urine. The crystals are round, occasionally with projections and brownish gold in color (50×).

- If the liver is unable to convert ammonia into urea, this will result in a severe accumulation of ammonia in the blood. Clinically, these patients can present with severe neurologic signs including head pressing, depression, and seizures.
- Ammonia can be measured but it must be measured immediately.
- Check with the laboratory running the test to determine if they need EDTA plasma or heparinized plasma. With most assays, the sample needs to be run within 30–60 minutes so the sample may need to be driven to the laboratory and sent on ice.
- Ammonium biurate crystals
    - Patients with portosystemic shunts or in liver failure that have decreased urea and elevated ammonia levels will start excreting ammonia biurate crystals in the urine (Figure 4.15).
    - This crystal indicates liver disease in most animals although Dalmations can produce these crystals normally.
- Bilirubinuria
    - Small amounts of bilirubin can be normal in canine urine; however, in other species, it is indicative of cholestatic disease and can precede a bilirubinuria.

Muscle

A. When muscle damage is assessed, it is usually skeletal muscle that is damaged or diseased. Several diseases result in significant elevations in muscle-associated analytes and they generally involve muscle necrosis, degeneration, or myositis.
B. Diagnostic testing
- Several enzymes are used to identify the presence of muscle damage.

- Creatine kinase (CK) is the most common. This is a cytosolic enzyme that leaks out when myocytes are damaged. CK has a short half-life and rises acutely with muscle injury and returns to normal quickly.
    - The enzyme is very sensitive and will increase if the patient receives an intramuscular injection or with extreme exercise.
    - The half-life of the enzyme is about 4 hours so values will often return to normal within 2–3 days after the insult.
- Aspartate aminotransferase
    - AST was discussed earlier in this chapter and can be used to assess liver damage. AST is not as tissue specific for muscle as CK and can be found in hepatocytes, myocytes, red blood cells, and many other tissues.
    - AST is a cytosolic enzyme similar to CK but has a longer half-life. It takes longer to appreciate an increase than CK and also takes longer to return to normal. Interpretation of AST should include evaluation of other analytes used to evaluate liver and muscle. For example, AST should be evaluated as part of a panel with CK, ALT, and ALP in dogs and cats or CK, SDH and ALP in horses and cattle.
- Lactate dehydrogenase (LDH)
    - This enzyme is found in the liver, muscle, and erythrocytes. A slight amount of hemolysis can result in elevations in LDH.
    - The combination of AST and CK are a better diagnostic combination for muscle disease than LDH.
- Other laboratory abnormalities
    - Myoglobin
        - This is a protein essential for transporting oxygen to muscle. Elevations in this protein are a specific indicator of muscle necrosis.
        - It does not discolor the plasma but will result in a brown discoloration of the urine and will react with the urine dipstick for blood, similar to hemoglobin. Refer to Chapter 5 for tests to differentiate myoglobin from hemoglobin.
    - Potassium
        - Myocytes are rich in potassium and massive muscle necrosis can result in mild elevations in potassium.

Pancreas

The pancreas is an organ with both endocrine (glandular) and exocrine (primarily production of digestive enzymes) functions. The exocrine function of this organ will be emphasized in this section. Inflammation of the pancreas or pancreatitis is not only a common diagnosis but also a diagnosis difficult to confirm.

A. Pancreatitis
- Primarily diagnosed in dogs and cats.
- The diagnosis requires a combination of supportive clinical evidence combined with clinical pathology testing and/or abdominal ultrasound.
- Diagnostic tests

- Enzymes may leak into the plasma during pancreatic injury resulting in increased serum activity. Amylase and lipase are the two most frequently measured enzymes.
- Amylase is not specific to the pancreas, it is also found in the small intestine and liver. It is an enzyme important in the digestion of sugars.
    - Hyperamylasemia can occur not only in patients with pancreatitis but also in animals with prerenal or renal azotemia, intestinal, and hepatobiliary diseases.
- Lipase is a little bit more specific to the pancreas and is a reasonable screening test for pancreatitis. It contributes to digestion of fat. Elevations of 3–5 times the reference range are supportive of pancreatitis. Smaller increases can be seen secondary to glucocorticoid administration or GI disease.
- Pancreatic lipase immunoreactivity is a test that is available for dogs (cPLI) and cats (fPLI). In cats, the test has been found to be both highly sensitive and specific but elevations in dogs have been associated with other diseases such as GI disease and hyperlipidemia. This test is available as a snap test (IDEXX) that can be done in hospital (Figure 4.16). The results are reported as normal or increased. To receive an actual number, samples can be submitted to the Gastrointestinal Laboratory at Texas A&M College of Veterinary Medicine: www.vetmed.tamu.edu/gilab/service/assay
- The test requires 0.5 mL of nonhemolyzed serum from a fasted patient.

B. Exocrine pancreatic insufficiency (EPI) is a disease in dogs. These animals lack enzymes necessary for digestion of fat. Consequently, affected animals have voluminous amounts of feces high in fat content.

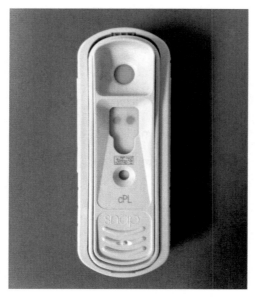

Figure 4.16   Results of a cPLI from a dog with suspected pancreatitis. The patient sample (top spot) is slightly darker than the control (bottom spot). If the patient sample is equally dark or darker than the control, this indicates a positive result.

- The best diagnostic test available is trypsin-like immunoreactivity (TLI). This assay detects trypsinogen and trypsin that are synthesized only by the pancreas. A decreased value is diagnostic for EPI.

Glucose

Glucose is a sugar that is used as an energy source for cellular metabolism. It is absorbed from the GI tract and is transported directly to the blood.

A. Sources of glucose
  - The primary source of glucose, particularly in young animals, is the diet. Neonates cannot go for long without eating because they can easily develop hypoglycemia.
  - Glycogenolysis
    - Glycogen is the main storage form of glucose in animals. Adult animals have abundant glycogen stores so it is unusual to see a healthy adult animal develop hypoglycemia secondary to anorexia. The process of glycogenolysis allows glycogen to be converted into glucose so it can be readily available to the cells. This process occurs primarily in the liver.
  - Gluconeogenesis is the production of glucose from amino acids and fat.
    - Glucocorticoids promote gluconeogenesis, which is one mechanism of hyperglycemia in stressed patients.
B. Utilization of glucose
  - Glycogenolysis
    - Glucose is stored as glycogen.
    - Glycogen synthesis occurs in the liver and skeletal muscle.
    - Glycogenolysis is promoted by insulin. Insulin is a hormone produced by the pancreas to allow cells to utilize glucose.
  - Glucose in tissue
    - Cellular uptake of glucose is mediated by insulin with the exception of red blood cells, neurons, and renal tubular epithelial cells.
    - The maintenance of blood glucose is a balancing act between insulin and insulin agonists.
C. Diagnostic tests
  - Blood glucose
    - This analyte is part of a general chemistry profile.
    - It can be measured on serum or plasma for most analyzers.
    - It is critical to centrifuge the sample as soon as possible and remove from the red blood cells or clot.
      - For serum, centrifuge as soon as the blood is clotted.
      - For plasma, centrifuge immediately.
      - Remove sample from the red blood cells immediately. If a serum separator tube is used, ensure that the gel has completely separated the serum from the clot (Figure 4.17).
    - If the red blood cells remain in contact with the serum or plasma, the cells will continue to metabolize glucose resulting in a false decrease in the patient's glucose level.

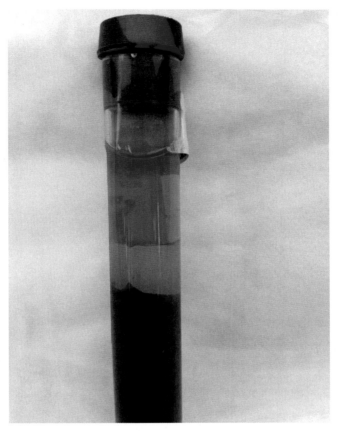

Figure 4.17   Blood from a dog, placed in a serum separation tube and centrifuged. The gel is completely separating the serum from the cells.

- Glucometer
  - Most glucometers use whole blood and only require a drop of blood.
    - There are many glucometers available so read the manufacturer's instructions on operation of the instrument.
  - The blood can be obtained from a sample drawn from a needle and syringe or an ear prick can be performed.
    - To perform an ear prick, shave a small area on the patient's ear, wipe with alcohol and with a 22 or 23 gauge needle, make a small prick in the ear. Take the glucose strip and hold it directly to the ear (Figure 4.18a–e).
- Urine glucose
  - Usually measured on a dipstick.
  - Diseases associated with glucosuria depend on the renal threshold for glucose. The renal threshold varies considerably in different species:
    - Cat ≈ 280 mg/dL
    - Dog ≈ 180 mg/dL
    - Horse ≈ 160 mg/dL
    - Cow ≈ 100 mg/dL

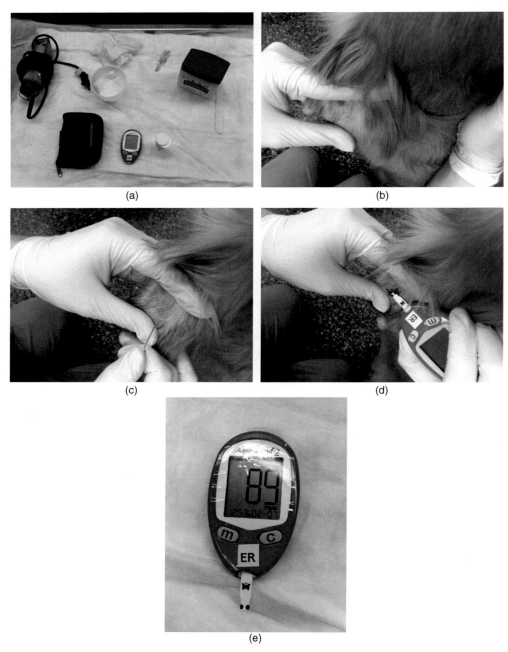

Figure 4.18   (a) Supplies needed to perform glucose measurement from an ear prick. (b) A small area of fur is shaved and sanitized to reveal the vein and safely puncture it with a needle. (c) The vein is punctured with the needle. (d) The test strip, appropriately inserted in the glucometer (follow the manufacturer instructions), is placed in the drop of blood. (e) The glucose level is determined by the glucometer and recorded in the patient's record.

- Stress (cortisol mediated) and fear (epinephrine mediated) can result in transient hyperglycemia and glucosuria. Fear and stress are more likely to result in glucosuria in the cow, horse and the dog due to the significantly lower renal threshold. However, excited or scared cats can exceed 280 mg/dL resulting in a transient glucosuria.
- Glycated proteins
  - Sugars bound to proteins, have a longer half-life, and will remain elevated for longer periods of time so that the clinician can differentiate hyperglycemia associated with fear from diseases causing a more persistent elevation in glucose-like diabetes mellitus.
    - Fructosamine is the most common glycated protein used in veterinary medicine.
    - Fructosamine is bound to albumin and the half-life of albumin is 1–2 weeks, therefore, if a patient that currently is hyperglycemic also has an elevated fructosamine, it suggests that the hyperglycemia is more than transient.
D. Diseases associated with hyperglycemia
  - Diabetes mellitus
    - Type I diabetes mellitus (decreased insulin production) and type II diabetes mellitus (delayed insulin secretion or inadequate insulin secretion) both can result in severe elevations in blood glucose or hyperglycemia.
    - Glucose levels can exceed 400–500 mg/dL.
    - It is a good idea to also check the urine for the presence of glucose and ketones.
  - Hyperadrenocorticism can be caused by a tumor of the adrenal gland or pituitary gland that produces excessive amounts of cortisol.
  - Transient hyperglycemia from fear or stress, pancreatitis, hyperthyroidism, or postprandial can also result in significant elevations in glucose.
E. Diseases associated with hypoglycemia or low levels of blood glucose
  - Neoplasms can induce hypoglycemia by several mechanisms by producing insulin or utilizing large amounts of glucose due to the increased metabolism and growth rate.
  - Hypoadrenocorticism
  - Hypothyroidism
  - Liver failure and portosystemic shunts
  - Young animals with anorexia
  - Sepsis
  - Inappropriate sample preparation
    - Delayed centrifugation
    - Sample left sitting on the clot
    - Gel in serum separator tube does not completely separate serum from clot.

Electrolytes

Electrolytes are minerals in the blood and body fluids that have an electrical charge and include calcium, phosphorus, sodium, potassium, and chloride. They are often grouped based on their function. Calcium and phosphorus are vital components of bone and other structural elements. Sodium, chloride, and potassium are all monovalent electrolytes important in fluid balance and are often discussed together.

Calcium

A. Calcium
- Functions
  - Calcium is a mineral that is a major structural contributor to bone and has many functions at the cellular level including ion gating across cell membranes, activation of cellular contraction, and secretion.
- Laboratory testing
  - Different forms of calcium are present in circulation, total, ionized, and complexed calcium.
  - Total calcium is a combination of ionized calcium, calcium bound to albumin, and calcium bound to nonprotein ions such as phosphate and lactate.
  - Measurement of total calcium
    - Approximately 40–50% of total calcium is bound to albumin.
    - Hypoalbuminemia can falsely decrease total calcium but will not affect ionized calcium.
    - The majority of in-house general chemistry analyzers will measure only total calcium.
  - Ionized calcium
    - Specialized analyzers will measure ionized calcium. This is a true reflection of the patient's functional calcium level.
B. Calcium to phosphorus ratio (Ca:P)
- Physiologically, this ratio is very important. Increases or decreases in calcium will affect phosphorus levels and vice versa.
- These minerals are controlled by hormones.
  - Parathyroid hormone (PTH) is produced by the parathyroid gland. Low serum calcium should result in an increased production of PTH. PTH increases calcium resorption from bone and absorption of calcium from the GI tract. It also increases excretion of phosphorus by the kidney.
  - Calcitonin is a hormone produced in the thyroid gland. If the calcium is increased, calcitonin is produced to decrease calcium absorption from the intestines, decrease calcium reabsorption from the renal tubules, and inhibit resorption of calcium from bones.
C. Hypercalcemia
- Primary hyperparathyroidism
  - If a patient has a tumor or hyperplastic tissue in the parathyroid gland, active, unregulated production of PTH can result in markedly elevated total and ionized calcium.
  - PTH levels can be measured in serum at specialty endocrine laboratories such as at Michigan State University, animalhealth.msu.edu
    - To measure PTH and ionized Ca^{2+}, 1 mL of serum is needed. Draw blood into a red top tube, let the sample clot for 30–60 minutes, centrifuge, and

remove the serum into a separate tube. Refrigerate or freeze the sample before sending to the laboratory.
- Pseudohyperparathyroidism (humoral hypercalcemia)
  - Some neoplastic cells can produce a protein similar to PTH called PTH-related peptide or PTH-rp. It has similar functions to PTH and can result in significant elevations in calcium.
  - Tumors that can produce PTH-rp include the following:
    - Lymphoma (T cell lymphoma)
    - Apocrine gland adenocarcinoma of the anal sac
    - Other carcinomas, less commonly
  - Laboratory abnormalities identified with humoral hypercalcemia include the following:
    - Marked increase in total calcium
    - Increased ionized calcium
    - Decreased phosphorus
    - Increased PTH-rp
    - Normal to decreased PTH
  - Other tumors can produce hypercalcemia by mechanisms other than PTH-rp. These tumors include the following:
    - Osteosarcoma
    - Multiple myeloma
    - Squamous cell carcinoma
    - Histiocytic sarcoma
    - Others
- Vitamin D toxicity
  - Vitamin D stimulates intestinal absorption of calcium, stimulates osteoclasts to respond to PTH and decreases excretion of calcium by the kidney. Osteoclasts are cells present in bone that have the ability to break down the mineralized component of bone and release calcium.
  - Several toxins can result in vitamin D toxicity, especially rodenticides containing cholecalciferol.
  - Laboratory abnormalities associated with vitamin D toxicity include the following:
    - Increased total and ionized calcium
    - Increased phosphorus
    - Decreased PTH
- Renal failure
  - Hypercalcemia secondary to renal disease is more common in horses because they excrete calcium via the kidneys. The decreased GFR associated with renal disease can result in hypercalcemia.
  - Rare in the dog and cat
- Hypoadrenocorticism (Addison's disease)
  - Mechanism of hypercalcemia is unknown.
D. Hypocalcemia (decreased calcium)
  - Decrease in total calcium

- Occurs most commonly with hypoalbuminemia but does not represent a true hypocalcemia because only the total calcium is decreased, the ionized calcium is normal.
- Primary hypoparathyroidism
  - Disease of the parathyroid glands resulting in inadequate PTH production in the face of hypocalcemia. Often secondary to surgery or trauma in the area of the gland.
  - Without PTH, there is decreased calcium resorption from bone, decreased absorption from the intestine, and decreased excretion of phosphorus by the kidney.
  - Laboratory abnormalities
    - Decreased total and ionized calcium
    - Increased phosphorus
    - Decreased PTH
- Renal secondary hyperparathyroidism
  - Renal failure impacts calcium and phosphorus metabolism in several ways.
    - In dogs and cats, phosphorus is excreted primarily through the kidneys. Decreased glomerular filtration with renal failure results in decreased excretion of phosphorus.
    - The kidneys play an important role in vitamin D metabolism, so in patients in renal failure, there is less active vitamin D.
    - These abnormalities result in increased PTH and secondary hyperparathyroidism.
- Nutrition
  - Animals with a vitamin D-deficient diet or decreased Ca:P can develop severe hypocalcemia. The name of this disease is called rickets.
- Milk fever
  - Occurs in cows in the peak of milk production (lactation)
    - The cow has an increased demand for calcium resulting in a severe, life-threatening hypocalcemia.
    - The hypocalcemia stimulates the production of PTH by the parathyroid glands.
    - Hypophosphatemia may also occur because of the increased renal excretion of phosphorus with increased production of PTH.
  - Other species can develop eclampsia with pregnancy. This too is a severe, life-threatening, hypocalcemia.
  - Cats can develop preparturient hypocalcemia 1–2 weeks before giving birth.
- Other causes of hypocalcemia include pancreatitis, ethylene glycol toxicity, certain diuretics, contamination of the sample with EDTA, and black widow spider envenomation.

TECHNICIAN TIP 4–3   Contamination of a serum sample with EDTA can result in severe hypocalcemia, sometimes as low as 1 or 2 mg/dL and depending on the type of EDTA, a marked elevation in potassium. If the EDTA tube is filled first and contacts the needle by inverting the tube to mix the blood, which small amount of contact is enough to contaminate the serum sample.

Phosphorus

A. Physiology
  - Phosphorus is an important component of adenosine triphosphate (ATP) and therefore essential for energy production.
  - Structural contributions are essential.
    - Phosphorus contributes to the structure of the matrix of bone, phosphoproteins, and phospholipids.
  - Calcium metabolism
    - The Ca:P ratio is essential for appropriate calcium metabolism. It is regulated by PTH, calcitriol, and calcitonin
B. Laboratory testing
  - Phosphorus can be tested on most chemistry analyzers.
C. Hyperphosphatemia
  - The most common cause of an elevated phosphorus or hyperphosphatemia is from decreased urinary excretion. This can occur secondarily to decreased GFR from prerenal or renal azotemia.
  - Hypoparathyroidism can cause hyperphosphatemia in addition to hypocalcemia. PTH induces an increase in urinary excretion of phosphorus. Therefore, in the absence of PTH, phosphorus will accumulate in the blood.
  - Young growing animals will have higher phosphorus levels compared to adults. This is a normal finding due to bone growth and metabolism.
  - Hypervitaminosis D will result in elevations in both phosphorus and calcium.
D. Hypophosphatemia
  - Increased renal excretion secondary to diuresis from fluid therapy or severe polydipsia.
  - Decreased intestinal absorption from anorexia or vitamin D deficiency.
  - Milk fever in cattle can cause a severe hypophosphatemia.
  - Renal failure in horses

Sodium, Chloride, and Potassium

A. Measurement of the electrolytes
  - If a sample is being sent out for analysis, the majority of the high volume chemistry analyzers and some in-house analyzers measure electrolytes with ion-specific electrodes that are fairly specific for each electrolyte. This technique is one of the best and can be performed on serum or plasma. If heparinized plasma is used, care must be taken not to use sodium heparin tubes for chemistry analysis. The sodium in the tube will significantly interfere with the assay.
B. Sodium (Na^+)
  - Physiologic functions
    - Sodium is the primary cation (positively charged substrate) in extracellular fluid. For that reason, it is vital for the movement of fluid and other electrolytes across epithelial barriers. Sodium is critical for the kidney to be able to reabsorb water from urine and concentrate the urine.

- Hyponatremia or decreased sodium usually occurs secondary to loss of sodium. Causes include the following:
  - Diarrhea
  - Urinary excretion
  - Sweating or salivating in the horse
  - Hypersalivation in cattle
  - Dilutional from diuresis either from intravenous or from subcutaneous fluids, psychogenic polydipsia, or administration of hypotonic fluids.
- Hypernatremia (elevated sodium) usually results from fluid loss consisting of pure water loss that can occur with diabetes insipidus, heat stress, and fever or a hypotonic fluid loss from diarrhea, vomiting, or chronic renal failure.

C. Chloride (Cl^-)
  - Physiologic functions
    - Chloride is the principal anion in extracellular fluid and accompanies sodium in order to maintain electric neutrality.
  - Hypochloremia often accompanies a hyponatremia and will decrease from similar mechanisms as sodium. Chloride can also be lost or sequestered without sodium. Examples of this include vomiting in dogs and cats, displaced abomasum in ruminants, and proximal duodenal obstruction.
  - Hyperchloremia with normal sodium can occur in patients with severe large bowel diarrhea or can be artificially elevated in patients being treated with potassium bromide therapy for seizures. The chloride and bromide are similar in structure and may be measured together.

D. Potassium (K^+)
  - Physiologic functions
    - Potassium is the principle cation for intracellular fluid. It is essential for cardiac rhythm and rate, renal sodium excretion and reabsorption, and acid–base metabolism.
  - Hypokalemia (decreased potassium)
    - There are three main mechanisms:
    - Decreased intake
      - Anorexia, especially in cattle, is a very common cause of hypokalemia.
    - Increased loss
      - Most likely from vomiting and/or diarrhea.
    - Redistribution between intracellular and extracellular fluid.
      - Glucose and insulin administration will drive the potassium into the cell.
  - Hyperkalemia
    - There are three main mechanisms:
      - Decreased urinary excretion
        - Can occur with hypoadrenocorticism, renal failure with accompanying decreased urine production, and urinary tract obstruction/ruptured urinary bladder.
      - Redistribution between the intracellular fluid and the extracellular fluid
        - Can be seen with metabolic acidosis.

- Artificial increases in potassium from hemolysis
  - Certain breeds of dogs (such as the Akita and Shiba Inu) and horses have increased amounts of intraerythrocytic potassium so if the red cells lyse, they release larger amounts of potassium than other animals.
  - Contamination with K^+ EDTA; EDTA contaminated samples will also have a markedly decreased calcium.
E. Sodium to potassium ratio (Na:K)
  - In healthy animals, this ratio is around 30. Increases in the ratio are not specific to any one disease because there are many nonspecific causes of hypokalemia.
  - The ratio can be easily calculated by dividing the sodium by the potassium. For example, a patient with a Na^+ of 140 and a K^+ of 4.0 will have a Na:K of 35.
  - A decreased Na:K can be clinically significant.
    - A ratio <23–25 is suggestive of several different diseases in dogs
      - Hypoadrenocorticism is a disease resulting from a malfunctioning adrenal cortex. The adrenal cortex produces mineralocorticoids, which are responsible for renal excretion of potassium and conservation of sodium. Patients with this disease can develop a severe hyperkalemia and hyponatremia.
      - Renal failure with decreased urine production can develop a severe hyperkalemia just due to decreased excretion of potassium.
      - Ruptured bladder with resulting uroperitoneum (urine in the abdomen). The urine contains high levels of potassium. When the urine is released in the abdomen, eventually all of the contents of the urine will be reabsorbed back into the blood causing a significant azotemia and hyperkalemia.
      - Other less common causes include whipworm infestation and repeated drainage of a chylothorax. These patients are more likely to have a hyponatremia with a normal potassium.

Acid–Base Balance

Serum electrolyte concentrations also contribute to the overall acid–base balance of the animal. Anions and cations in an animal are balanced to maintain the pH of the blood at a neutral level (neither acidic nor basic). The pH of a healthy animal should be between 7.35 and 7.45. If the pH of the blood is less than 7.35, the patient is considered acidemic. If the pH is greater than 7.45, the patient is considered alkalemic. In addition to the pH, many different analytes are measured or calculated in determination of the patient's acid–base status. Thorough evaluation of acid–base includes three inter-related components: blood gas, serum electrolytes, and anion gap.

A. Blood gas analysis
  - Arterial or venous blood can be sampled to analyze a blood gas.
  - The components of the blood gas consist of partial pressures of oxygen (pO_2) and carbon dioxide (pCO_2), pH, bicarbonate (HCO^{3-}), oxygen saturation of blood, and base excess.
  - Sample preparation

- Whole blood is analyzed, usually heparinized. A small amount of heparin is added to the syringe by aspirating heparin in the syringe to coat the syringe and then expelling the heparin. The sample type is the same or arterial or venous blood.
- The sample should be measured immediately, especially an arterial sample. After the blood is drawn from the patient, the needle should be capped with a rubber stopper or cork. If the sample cannot be analyzed immediately, it should be placed on ice and analyzed within 30 minutes.
- Blood gas analytes
  - pO_2: Measures the ability of the lungs to oxygenate the blood. This analyte is most commonly measured in arterial blood rather than venous. A decrease in oxygen level in the blood is referred to as hypoxia. Causes of hypoxia can include primary lung disease such as pneumonia, impaired ventilation such as hypoventilation with anesthesia, and inhaling atmosphere with decreased oxygen as seen at high altitudes.
  - pCO_2: This is the partial pressure of carbon dioxide in the blood. $PaCO_2$, in the arterial blood, is an excellent reflection of respiratory ventilation. In this case, the "a" indicates that the sample was taken from an artery rather than a vein. The reference range of $PaCO2$ is 35–45 mmHg.
  - pH: This is the concentration of hydrogen ions in the blood. The normal pH of blood is 7.35-7.45. An increase of the pH is alkalemia and a decrease in the pH is acidemia. The kidney helps control the pH by regulating the retention and excretion of HCO^{3-}. The respiratory system also helps control the blood pH by regulating the expulsion of $pCO2$ through the respiratory rate.
  - HCO^{3-}: Bicarbonate is responsible for buffering the blood and increasing the blood pH when increased acids such as lactic acid or uremic acids are present. As mentioned earlier, bicarbonate is conserved or secreted by the kidneys to help maintain acid–base regulation. Increased amounts of bicarbonate result in metabolic alkalosis and decreased bicarbonate results in metabolic acidosis.
  - Base excess (BE): This is determined through a calculation using bicarbonate, hemoglobin, $pCO2$, and body temperature. The BE should equal $0+/-3$ mEq/L. An increased BE indicates a metabolic alkalosis and a decreased BE indicates a metabolic acidosis.
- Acid–base analytes from the chemistry profile
  - Total carbon dioxide ($tCO2$) effectively is the equivalent of bicarbonate. $tCO2$ is the total gas released when a serum or plasma sample is mixed with a strong acid. 95% of $tCO2$ is bicarbonate.
  - Anion gap is also a calculation. The equation is $(Na^++K^+)-(Cl^-+HCO_3^-)$. It is used to detect the presence of unmeasured anions or cations. In patients with metabolic acidosis, the anion gap can be used to help determine the cause of the acidosis. An increased anion gap will occur if there are unmeasured anions such as ketones, lactic acid, uremic acids, or metabolites of toxins such as ethylene glycol. A decreased anion gap is much less common but indicates the presence of unmeasured cations. It can be seen in patients with severe hypoalbuminemia.

Table 4.4   Summary of acid–base disorders and typical blood gas changes.

Disorder	pH	HCO^{3-}/tCO$_2$	pCO$_2$
Metabolic acidosis (uncompensated)	D	D	N
Metabolic acidosis (partial compensation)	D	D	D
Metabolic alkalosis (uncompensated)	I	I	N
Metabolic alkalosis (partial compensation)	I	I	I
Respiratory acidosis (uncompensated)	D	N	I
Respiratory acidosis (partial compensation)	D	I	I
Respiratory alkalosis (uncompensated)	I	N	D
Respiratory alkalosis (partial compensation)	I	D	D

D = decreased
I = Increased
N = Normal or no change

- Acid–base disturbances
  - The first step to evaluating an acid–base disturbance is identifying an increase or decrease in the pH. If the pH is decreased, the patient has an acidosis. If the pH is increased, there is an alkalosis. The next step is to try to identify the cause of the disturbance as metabolic or respiratory.
  - Metabolic acidosis is characterized by a decreased blood pH and decreased bicarbonate or tCO2.
    - Metabolic acidosis can occur with a decrease in bicarbonate-rich fluids such as diarrhea, loss of bicarbonate in the urine (renal tubular acidosis), and in ruminants, excessive loss of saliva. Laboratory abnormalities will include decreased tCO2 or bicarbonate and decreased sodium and chloride and normal anion gap.
    - A metabolic acidosis can also occur when bicarbonate is used to titrate excessive acids. This is called a titrational metabolic acidosis. Bicarbonate acts as a buffer and it is converted into the salt of the acid, which results in an increased anion gap. Patients with lactic acidosis, uremic acids, and ketones can develop this type of acidosis. Laboratory abnormalities with a titrational metabolic acidosis include decreased pH, decreased bicarbonate, and increased anion gap.
  - Metabolic alkalosis is characterized by an increased blood pH and elevated bicarbonate. Metabolic alkalosis occurs most commonly in dogs and cats that are vomiting. The stomach is rich in hydrochloric acid (HCl). The loss of this acidic fluid results in an elevation in bicarbonate in the blood. Ruminants have four chambers to their stomach. The abomasum is the equivalent to the stomach of the dog and cat. If the abomasum is displaced or torsed, HCl will get sequestered in the abomasum and the patient will develop a significant metabolic alkalosis. Laboratory abnormalities in vomiting or displaced abomasum include elevated bicarbonate and decreased chloride.

- Respiratory acidosis is not very common but can occur with decreased respiratory ventilation. Laboratory abnormalities include a decreased pH and elevated pCO2. Patients with severe pulmonary disease or abnormal ventilation during anesthesia can develop respiratory acidosis. No abnormalities will be seen on the chemistry profile, a blood gas analysis is necessary to diagnose this abnormality.
- Respiratory alkalosis occurs in patients with increased respiratory ventilation or increased respiratory rate. Blood gas abnormalities in these patients include an increased pH and decreased pCO2. Dogs that are panting excessively can develop respiratory alkalosis.
- Compensation
  - As an acid–base abnormality develops, the patient will attempt to compensate. If there is a metabolic disturbance, the respiratory system attempts to compensate. For example, if the patient has a metabolic acidosis, the patient will attempt to correct the pH by eliminating pCO2 and increasing its respiratory rate. If there is a respiratory acid–base disturbance, there is metabolic compensation. The kidney will attempt to retain or excrete bicarbonate to compensate for the primary disturbance. Metabolic compensation can take several days to begin, whereas respiratory compensation can occur immediately (Table 4.4).

Further Reading

Bauer J.E., Harvey J.W., Asquith R.L., et al. (1985) Serum protein reference values in foals during the first year of life: comparison of chemical and electrophoretic methods. *Veterinary Clinical Pathology*, 14(1), 14–22.

Berent A.C, Murakami T., Scroggin R.D., et al. (2005) Reliability of using reagent test strips to estimate blood urea nitrogen concentration in dogs and cats. *Journal of the American Veterinary Medical Association*, 227(8), 1253–1256.

Bishop, M.L., Duben-VonLaufen, J.L. & Fody, E.P. (eds.) (1985). *Clinical Chemistry Principles, Procedures, Correlations*. Philadelphia, PA: J.B. Lippincott Company.

Cortadellas O., Fernandez del Palacio M.J., Talavera J., *et al.* (2010) Calcium and phosphorus homeostasis in dogs with spontaneous chronic kidney disease at different stages of severity. *Journal Veterinary Internal Medicine*, 24, 73–79.

Center S.A., Baldwin B.H., Dillingham S., *et al.* (1986) Diagnostic value of serum γ-glutamyl transferase and alkaline phosphatase activities in hepatobiliary disease in the cat. *Journal of the American Veterinary Medical Association*, 188(5), 507–510.

Ettinger, S.J. & Feldman, E.C., (eds) (2010). *Textbook of Veterinary Internal Medicine* (7th ed.). St. Louis, MO: Saunders Elsevier.

Fernandez N.J. & Kidney B.A. (2007) Alkaline phosphatase: beyond the liver. *Veterinary Clinical Pathology*, 36(3), 223–233.

Foreman M.A., Marks S.L., De Cock H.E., *et al.* (2004) Evaluation of the serum feline pancreatic lipase immunoreactivity and helical computed tomography versus conventional testing for the diagnosis of feline pancreatitis. *Journal Veterinary Internal Medicine*, 18(6), 807–815.

Gaskill C.L., Miller L.M., Mattoon J.S., *et al.* (2005) Liver histopathology and liver and serum alanine aminotransferase and alkaline phosphatase activities in epileptic dogs receiving phenobarbital. *Veterinary Pathology*, 42, 147–160.

Harison E., Langston C., Palma D., *et al.* (2012) Acute azotemia as a predictor of mortality in dogs and cats. *Journal Veterinary Internal Medicine*, 26, 1093–1098.

Israeli I., Steiner J., Segev G., *et al.* (2012) Serum pepsinogen-A, canine pancreatic lipase immunoreactivity, and C-reactive protein as prognostic markers in dogs with gastric dilatation-volvulus. *Journal Veterinary Internal Medicine*, 26(4), 920–928.

Jacob F., Polzin D.J., Osborne C.A., et al. (2005) Evaluation of the association between initial proteinuria and morbidity rate or death in dogs with naturally occurring chronic renal failure. *Journal of the American Veterinary Medical Association*, 226(3), 393–400.

Kalaitzakis E., Roubies N., Panousis N., *et al.* (2007) Clinicopathologic evaluation of hepatic lipidosis in periparturient dairy cattle. *Journal Veterinary Internal Medicine*, 21, 835–845.

Latimer, K.S. (ed) (2011) *Duncan & Prasse's Veterinary Laboratory Medicine Clinical Pathology*, 5th edn. Wiley-Blackwell, Ames, IA.

Neel J.A. & Grindem C.B.. (2000) Understanding and evaluating renal function. *Veterinary Medicine*, 95, 555–566.

Nestor D.D., Holan K.M., Johnson C.A., *et al.* (2006) Serum alkaline phosphatase activity in Scottish Terriers versus dogs of other breeds. *Journal of the American Veterinary Medical Association*, 228(2), 222–224.

Prause L.C. & Grauer G.F.. (1998) Association of gastrointestinal hemorrhage with increased blood urea nitrogen and BUN/creatinine ratio in dogs: a literature review and retrospective study. *Veterinary Clinical Pathology*, 27(4), 107–111.

Sepesy L.M., Center S.A., Randolph J.F., *et al.* (2006) Vacuolar hepatopathy in dogs: 336 cases (1993–2005). *Journal of the American Veterinary Medical Association*, 229(2), 246–252.

Stockham, S.L., & Scott, M.A. (2008). *Fundamentals of Veterinary Clinical Pathology* (2nd ed.). Ames, IA: Blackwell Publishing.

Verkest K.R., Fleeman L.M., Morton J.M., *et al.* (2012) Association of postprandial serum triglyceride concentration and serum canine pancreatic lipase immunoreactivity in overweight and obese dogs. *Journal Veterinary Internal Medicine*, 26(1), 46–53.

Thrall, M.A., Weiser, G., Allison, R.W., & Campbell, T.W. (eds) (2012). *Veterinary Hematology and Clinical Chemistry*. Ames, IA: Wiley-Blackwell.

Xenoulis P.G., Suchodolski J.S., Levinski M.D., *et al.* (2008) Serum liver enzyme activities in healthy Miniature Schnauzers with and without hypertriglyceridemia. *Journal of the American Veterinary Medical Association*, 232(1), 63–67.

Zimmerman K.L., Panciera D.L., Panciera R.J., *et al.* (2010) Hyperphosphatasemia and concurrent adrenal gland dysfunction in apparently healthy Scottish Terriers. *Journal of the American Veterinary Medical Association*, 237(2), 178–186.

Activities

Multiple Choice Questions

1. Which erroneous result can occur with EDTA contamination?
   A) Hypokalemia
   B) Hypocalcemia
   C) Hypophosphatemia
   D) Hyponatremia

2. White, cloudy serum is suggestive of:
   A) Hemolysis
   B) Icterus
   C) Lipemia
   D) Contamination with anticoagulant

3. The presence of icteric serum indicates:
   A) Elevated total bilirubin
   B) Anemia
   C) Traumatic blood draw
   D) Increased lipid content

4. Hyperglobulinemia can occur with:
   A) Severe inflammation
   B) Diarrhea
   C) Hemorrhage
   D) Liver failure

5. A refractometer is used to measure:
   A) Electrolytes
   B) Enzymes
   C) Protein
   D) Lipemia

6. The presence of azotemia can occur with all EXCEPT:
   A) Dehydration
   B) Renal failure
   C) Ruptured bladder
   D) Psychogenic polydipsia

7. Which is commonly seen in patients with renal failure?
   A) Hyperphosphatemia
   B) Hyperglobulinemia
   C) Elevated ALT
   D) Elevated total bilirubin

8. Which enzyme indicates cholestatic disease?
   A) ALT
   B) ALP
   C) SDH
   D) AST

9. Which is NOT a pseudofunction test of the liver?
   A) Albumin
   B) Cholesterol
   C) Sodium
   D) Urea

10. Which enzyme is used to evaluate muscle disease?
    A) CK
    B) ALP
    C) Lipase
    D) GGT

Urinalysis

Anne M. Barger
University of Illinois, Champaign, IL, USA

Learning Objectives

1. The student should be able to perform a thorough urinalysis including urine chemistry, specific gravity, and sediment examination.
2. Have a basic understanding of renal physiology.
3. Understand the significance of the different cells within the urine sediment.
4. Be able to recognize common cells, crystals, and microorganisms.
5. Understand the limitations of each method of urine collection.

Case example 1

A 5-year-old spayed female poodle presents with a history of urinating in the house. The owner is concerned because the urine is red. The owner brought a urine sample she had collected at home. What could the red color of the urine indicate?

Answer: Red blood cells (hematuria) or hemoglobin (hemoglobinuria).

Clinical Pathology and Laboratory Techniques for Veterinary Technicians, First Edition.
Edited by Anne Barger and Amy MacNeill.
© 2015 John Wiley & Sons, Inc. Published 2015 by John Wiley & Sons, Inc.
Companion Website: www.wiley.com/go/barger/vettechclinpath

Case example 2

A 10-year-old, neutered male Dalmation presents for his annual physical examination. Blood and urine are collected for a senior wellness panel. Ammonium birurate crystals are identified in the urine sediment. What is the significance of these crystals in this patient?
Answer: None, they can be normal in this breed of dog. In other breeds, these crystals can indicate severe liver disease.

Introduction

A *urinalysis* is a series of diagnostic tests used primarily to evaluate kidney and overall urinary tract disease but also, as will be discussed in this chapter, some endocrine diseases and acid–base balance. It is an inexpensive test to perform and can easily be performed in the clinic setting. The purpose of this chapter is to describe the diagnostic tests used to fully interpret any abnormalities in the urine. A basic understanding of urine production is essential to understand why certain diagnostic tests are performed. A full urinalysis involves gross evaluation, measurement of the *specific gravity*, urine dipstick, and microscopic evaluation of the *urine sediment*. A urinalysis is considered a "screening" test because abnormal results will likely be followed up with another test or used in conjunction with serum chemistry results. This chapter begins with urine production and describes the tests used to fully evaluate urine.

Urine Production

The kidneys are paired organs responsible for fluid homeostasis, maintenance of acid–base balance, maintenance of electrolyte balance, and excretion of waste products. The activities of thousands of nephrons contribute to renal function. The components of the nephron include the glomerulus, proximal tubule, loop of Henle, distal tubule, and the collecting duct which empties into the renal medulla (Figure 5.1). Urine production is the combination of glomerular filtration, tubular reabsorption, and tubular secretion.

A. Glomerular filtration
   - This process is the filtration of blood from the glomerular capillaries into Bowman's capsule. The filtrate consists of a large amount of fluid, free of protein. Substrates other than protein are freely filtered. As fluid passes on to the tubules, water and solutes are reabsorbed or secreted depending on the physiologic state of the patient. The glomerular filter consists of endothelium from the capillaries, a basement membrane, and epithelial cells called podocytes. All three of these layers have a negative charge which helps repel protein.
B. Tubular reabsorption
   - Transport of material across the tubular epithelial membranes in the renal interstitial fluid occurs through the peritubular capillary membrane back into the blood and can be active or passive. Active transport requires energy derived

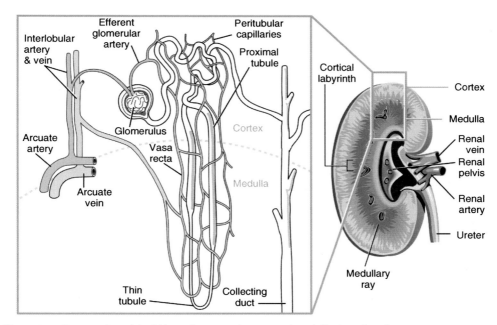

Figure 5.1   Cross section of the kidney shows renal cortex and medulla. Inset box demonstrates components of the nephron including glomerulus, proximal renal tubule, and collecting duct.

from metabolism of adenosine triphosphate (ATP) or an ion gradient. Passive transport occurs by osmosis or electrical potential. The passive reabsorption of water is coupled primarily to sodium reabsorption. As sodium is transported out of the tubule, their concentration will decrease inside the tubule while increasing outside the cell. This creates a concentration gradient so water can then follow sodium.

C. Tubule specifics
  - Proximal tubule
    - The majority of sodium, water, and chloride are reabsorbed here with a very high capacity for active and passive reabsorption.
  - Loop of Henle
    - Has two parts, the thin descending limb where water and urea are freely filtered and the thick ascending limb that relies on active transport for reabsorption sodium and chloride.
  - Distal tubule
    - Sodium, chloride, and potassium are avidly reabsorbed here but the distal tubule is impermeable to urea and water.
  - Collecting duct
    - Requires the action of antidiuretic hormone (ADH) to absorb water.
D. Tubular secretion
  - Tubular secretion is the active release of substances by the tubular epithelial cells into the lumen of the nephron. This is useful to maintain electrolyte balances, primarily in the secretion of potassium, and the maintenance of acid–base balance with secretion of hydrogen ion.

Concentration of Urine

The kidney functions to conserve water in a dehydrated patient and to excrete water in a patient that is well hydrated. The kidneys rely on the concentrating ability of the nephron to conserve water. Dilute urine forms by continually reabsorbing solute from the urine so even kidneys with dilute urine have functional nephrons.

- Concentration of urine requires two very specific criteria:
  - A high level of ADH which will increase permeability of the distal tubules and collecting ducts to water.
  - High osmolarity of the renal medullary interstitial fluid which provides the osmotic gradient necessary for water reabsorption to occur in the presence of ADH (hypertonic medulla).
- How does the renal medulla become hypertonic?
  - There is an accumulation of solutes in the renal medulla, primarily sodium and urea.
  - Sodium is actively reabsorbed from the ascending loop of Henle along with chloride. The process of reabsorption of sodium and urea happens over and over again, eventually resulting in a hypertonic medulla. This process is referred to as the countercurrent multiplier. Sodium and urea are critical for the kidney to concentrate urine.
  - Urea is reabsorbed in the proximal tubule. The thick limb of the loop of Henle, distal tubule, and cortical collecting duct are impermeable to urea. The inner medullary collecting duct is permeable to urea which diffuses into the medullary interstitium.
  - Patients with hyponatremia and decreased urea may have a hypotonic medulla, resulting in medullary washout and an inability of the kidney to concentrate the urine.
- Urine concentration conclusions:
  - Urine is concentrated by reabsorbing water
  - ADH, functioning nephrons, and a hypertonic renal medulla are essential to this process.
  - Urine is diluted by reabsorbing solute.
  - Functional nephrons are essential for this process (Table 5.1).

Urine Collection

Urine collection should be done before any therapy which would include fluid and drug administration. This will allow for the best interpretation of the kidney function and diagnosis of disease. Urine can be collected by several different methods and each has limitations.

A. Free catch/voided sample
   - Advantages of free catch include no risk of trauma and the owners can bring in a sample, provided they have placed it in a clean container. Disadvantages include possible sample contamination by the patient and or environment and

Table 5.1   Summary of osmolarity and concentrating ability of tubules.

1. Proximal Tubule: Absorption of NaCl and water
2. Descending loop of Henle: Highly permeable to water but less permeable to NaCl and urea
3. Thin ascending limb of the loop of Henle: Impermeable to water but allows reabsorption of NaCl
4. Thick ascending limb of the loop of Henle: Abundant absorption of NaCl, minimal absorption of water
5. Early distal tubule: Solute reabsorption
6. Late distal tubule and cortical collecting duct: ADH

ADH: permeable to water ADH: impermeable to water
*Impermeable to urea so when water in reabsorbed, urine becomes concentrated.
Most of urea is delivered to medullary collecting ducts to be absorbed or is passed
into urine.

patient compliance is essential. Free catch samples will not be sterile because the urine passes through many structures before leaving the patient. The distal urethra, vagina, and in male dogs prepuce are not sterile, and therefore, a voided urine specimen is not ideal for culture.
- Mid-stream collection is ideal because this will limit contamination from the patient. Initial stream will likely have greater numbers of cells and microorganisms from the prepuce which are flushed and often limited in the midstream.
- Cats are more challenging to collect urine from as a free catch. Removal of litter from the litter box or use of non-absorbable litter often is necessary.
B. Manual expression
- This can be very traumatic to the patient and if the patient has underlying disease of the bladder, it may result in serious bladder injury. In addition, the urine is subject to the same level of contamination as a free catch. This method is no longer recommended unless urine cannot be collected by any other method.
C. Urinary catheterization
- Urinary catheterization can be a method to collect urine for diagnostic testing and can also be used to relieve urinary obstruction and as a method to measure urinary output.
- Some disadvantages include mucosal damage and secondary infection. Urinary catheterization must be performed with sterility.
D. Cystocentesis
- This technique is the best for collecting urine for culture. Urine in the bladder of healthy animals should be sterile so any bacteria cultured from these samples are likely from the bladder.
- Cystocentesis is performed by palpating and stabilizing the bladder and inserting a needle into the bladder and removing urine with an attached syringe (Figure 5.2). A small gauge needle (e.g., a 22 gauge needle) is ideal and less

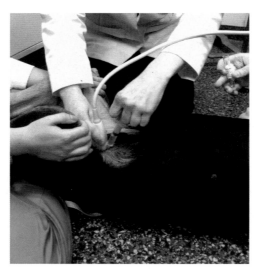

Figure 5.2   Ultrasound guidance is demonstrated to assist in directing the needle into the bladder. The needle is attached to the syringe, inserted in the urinary bladder, and urine is aspirated.

Table 5.2   Advantages and disadvantages of different methods of urine collection.

	Advantage	Disadvantage
Free catch	Ease of collection	Contamination with bacteria limits use of this sample for culture
Manual collection	Not recommended	Traumatic to the patient
Catheterization	If sterile technique is used, the sample may be used for culture	Mucosal damage and risk of iatrogenic secondary infection
Cystocentesis	Best sample for culture	Blood contamination is common so this technique is not ideal for evaluation of urine protein Special training is required to perform this technique

traumatic for the patient. If the bladder is not palpable, ultrasound guidance may be used to assist in obtaining a sample.
• Disadvantages of cystocentesis are that patient cooperation is critical, blood contamination is common, and there is a slight risk of rupture/abdominal contamination especially if the patient has a urinary obstruction (Table 5.2).

Examination of Urine

A. General concepts
  • Urine should be examined as soon as possible. This will limit bacterial growth. The pH can change due to urease splitting bacteria. In addition, the urine is a

harsh environment and cells begin to autolyze fairly quickly. If the urine cannot be evaluated immediately, refrigeration is best; however, this can induce crystal formation in some samples.

> **TECHNICIAN TIP 5–1**   Evaluation of urine immediately will provide the most reliable results.

B. Gross examination
- Thorough gross examination is required to evaluate the color, clarity, and smell, which are important aspects of urine to evaluate. Abnormalities in any or all of these aspects indicate underlying pathology.
- Color
  - Normal urine is yellow: due to urochrome and urobilin (Figure 5.3a).
  - Red urine: due to red blood cells or hemoglobin (Figure 5.3a).
    - If intact red blood cells are present, the sample will clear with centrifugation.

> **TECHNICIAN TIP 5–2**   Red urine can be centrifuged. If the red color is eliminated, hematuria is the likely cause of the discoloration.

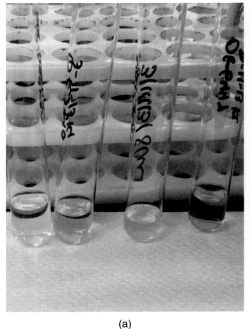
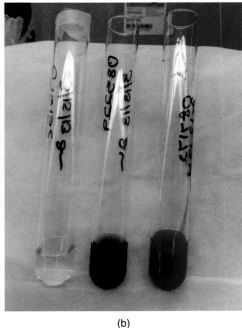

(a)   (b)

Figure 5.3   (a and b) Urine from different dogs demonstrating yellow, red, and brown urine. The red urine in this image contained many red blood cells, and the brown urine contained 4+ bilirubin.

- Dark yellow to brown: indicates bilirubin (Figure 5.3b).
- Reddish brown: due to hemoglobin or myoglobin. Myoglobin is a pigment from muscle damage and can be seen in horses with rhabdomyolysis or dogs with severe seizures or other muscle trauma.
  - Clarity
    - Normal urine should be clear. In most species, if you hold a sample in a clear plastic or glass tube over printed text, you should be able to read the text clearly (Figure 5.4a). Any cloudiness in the urine indicates an "active" sediment with or without a pathologic sediment (Figure 5.4b). The exception to this is equine urine. Owing to the presence of crystals and mucous, their urine is usually cloudy.
    - Causes of increased turbidity include cells, primarily white and red blood cells, crystals, mucus, bacteria, casts, and sperm.
  - Odor
    - Normal urine has an aroma; however, there are some pathological changes that can result in atypical odor.
      - Ammonia can be detected in normal feline urine but in other species, this odor may be suggestive of liver disease.
      - Excessive protein breakdown
      - Ketonuria gives urine a very sweet odor. Not all individuals can detect the smell of ketones in the urine.

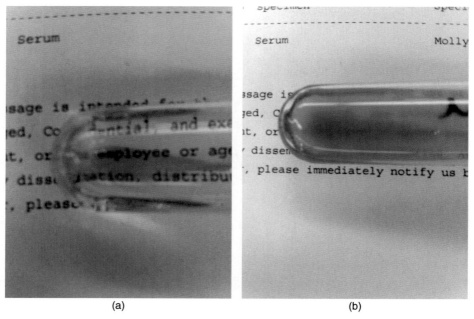

(a)   (b)

Figure 5.4 (a) Urine with an inactive sediment should be clear, so clear that print can be easily read through the urine. Note the clarity of the letters through the urine. (b) Urine with an active sediment (containing crystals, cells, bacteria, etc.) is more likely to be cloudy and can easily visualized by holding the urine over printed text. Note how difficult it is to read the text through the urine in this sample.

Urine Concentration

A. Urine-specific gravity
  - This is the most common method of determining the functioning capacity of the nephrons. The urine-specific gravity (USG) is the ratio of the weight of a volume of urine compared to the weight of the same volume of pure water. It is an indication of the concentration of dissolved material in the urine and is a reflection of the diluting and concentrating ability of the kidneys. The specific gravity of urine from healthy animals can be influenced by several factors including eating and drinking habits, environmental temperature, and when the sample was collected (first thing in the morning versus later in the day after the patient has had open access to water).
  - A refractometer can be used to determine the USG but it should be one equipped with the USG scale. The refractometer should be calibrated with water before use with urine. The specific gravity of water is 1.000. To use the refractometer with urine, 1 drop of urine is placed on the glass surface of the refractometer with the plastic cover closed and the urine is wicked to cover the glass surface via capillary action (Figure 5.5). The refractometer is then held up to a light source. Read the specific gravity where light meets dark on the USG scale (Figure 5.6). This is usually a clear demarcation. Most refractometers will only measure specific gravity to 1.035 so if it is greater than that, an aliquot of urine can be diluted with an equal amount of deionized water and measured again. The actual specific gravity can then be calculated by multiplying the decimal of the specific gravity measurement by the dilution factor and adding 1. For example, if the urine is diluted by adding 1 mL of water to 1 mL of urine (this is a 1:2 dilution) and the specific gravity of the diluted urine is 1.030, the actual specific gravity is calculated by multiplying the decimal of the USG by the

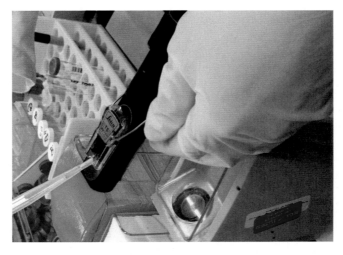

Figure 5.5   Urine is loaded into the refractometer by placing urine between the glass and the plastic cover.

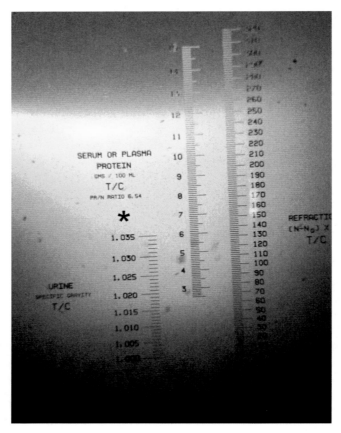

Figure 5.6 The scale labeled with an * is used to measure the urine-specific gravity. If the specific gravity is high (>1.035), urine may need to be diluted to obtain an accurate value.

dilution factor, in this case, 2. Therefore, the actual specific gravity in this example would be 1.060.

- The specific gravity of water is 1.000. The USG of urine should be greater than this. There is a normal wide range of 1.001–1.065. In cats, the USG can go as high as 1.080.
- *Hyposthenuria* indicates that the USG is quite low, <1.008. The specific gravity of the glomerular filtrate is 1.008–1.010, so hyposthenuric urine indicates that the kidney has an issue with concentration which could be as simple as a dog with polydipsia (increased water consumption) or a more severe endocrine disease such as hyperadrenocorticism.
- *Isosthenuria* indicates that the USG is 1.008–1.012, essentially unchanged from the glomerular filtrate. This USG is concerning if the patient is dehydrated. The clinical assessment of the patient, along with serum chemistry is critical when evaluating the USG. Isosthenuria can occur in patients with renal failure when >66% of the nephrons are nonfunctional.

Table 5.3   Summary of alterations in urine-specific gravity.

Elevated USG	Decreased USG
Dehydration	Increased fluid intake or administration
Decreased water intake	
Extreme heat	Psychogenic polydipsia
Shock	Hyperadrenocorticism

- Hypersthenuria is a term used to indicate an elevated USG and may occur if the patient is dehydrated. This term is not used commonly.
- Interpretation of urine concentration
  - Hydration status and clinical presentation of the patient are essential for correct interpretation of the USG.
    - An azotemic animal with inappropriately concentrated urine may be in renal failure (Table 5.3).
B. Urine volume
  - The amount of urine a patient is producing is very helpful in evaluation of the overall disease process.
  - *Polyuria* is a term used to indicate an increase in urine volume.
    - Polyuria can occur in patients with increased water consumption or receiving fluids and with corticosteroid therapy.
    - Diseases that can result in polyuria include acute or chronic renal failure, diabetes mellitus, diabetes insipidus, pyometra, hyperadrenocorticism, and many more.
  - *Oliguria* is used to describe decreased urine production.
    - Oliguria can occur with an increased environmental temperature or hyperventilation.
    - Pathologic causes of oliguria include dehydration, fever, acute, or end stage chronic renal failure and shock.
  - *Anuria* indicates that the patient is producing almost no urine and is always associated with disease.
    - Diseases that can result in anuria include urinary obstruction and toxic nephrosis. Causes of toxic nephrosis include ethylene glycol toxicity and arsenic.

Urine Chemistry

A. Urine chemistry can be measured on a urine dipstick (Figure 5.7). The dipsticks are simple to use. Briefly, dip the test pads completely in fresh, well-mixed urine, and remove quickly. Make sure that all test pads have been fully immersed in urine. Turn the test strip on its side on a paper towel or other absorbent paper to remove excess urine (Figure 5.8). At the appropriate times, compare the test pads with the chart on the dipstick container and record the results. It is ideal to perform these

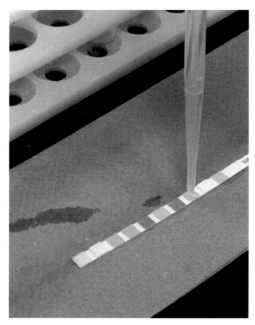

Figure 5.7   Urine is placed on the urine dipstick with either a pipet as pictured here or the urine can be literally "dipped" in the urine. The dipstick is evaluated after the time specified by the manufacturer by comparing the dipstick to a color-coded chart on the dipstick canister.

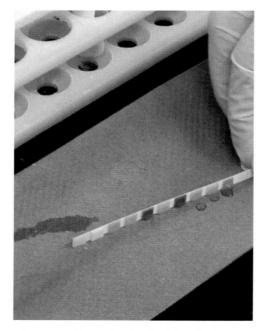

Figure 5.8   Excess urine can be removed by turning the dipstick on its side on a paper towel and gently tapping the excess urine onto the paper towel.

tests using uncentrifuged urine. However if the patient has marked hematuria, the sample may need to be centrifuged before chemical evaluation.

B. Specific tests on the urine dipstick
- Leukocyte
  - This is a human-specific assay. The test detects a specific antigen on human white blood cells. This test is not useful in veterinary medicine and does not cross-react with most species of animals. The urine sediment should be evaluated to identify white blood cells.
- pH (H^+ concentration)
  - Carnivores and omnivores (dogs and cats) have acidic urine and herbivores (ruminants and horses) have alkaline urine. It is important to understand what is normal for a species before trying to interpret the results.
  - Abnormal pH can indicate an acid–base abnormality, cystitis with urea splitting bacteria or be greatly impacted by therapy or diet.
- Glucose
  - Urine from healthy animals should be negative for glucose. The kidney has a threshold for glucose reabsorption. When this is exceeded, the patient starts to excrete glucose in the urine. The renal threshold varies considerably with species. In dogs, it is 180 mg/dL, cats have a much higher threshold at 280 mg/dL and cattle are much lower, <100 mg/dL.
  - *Glucosuria* can be seen in excited or scared animals, particularly cats or in patients that are chronically stressed. Diseases that result in marked hyperglycemia can consequently have glucosuria. These include diabetes mellitus and hyperadrenocorticism.
  - False positives can occur with patients receiving certain antibiotics such as cephalexin and enrofloxacin.
- Ketones
  - Normal urine is negative.
  - The test pad will turn purple when positive for ketones. A red, pink, or brown color change is not indicative of a positive test result.
  - Positive results can occur with starvation, particularly in young animals, diabetes mellitus, bovine ketosis, ovine pregnancy toxemia, a high fat diet, and secondary to severe vomiting and diarrhea.
  - Many test strips react with the ketones, acetone, and acetoacetone but are insensitive to b-hydroxybutyric acid (most common ketone in dogs and cats).
  - False results
    - False positive results can occur in calves with polioencephalomalacia and a false negative result can occur in old urine or with expired test strips. It is important to always use fresh urine and make sure that the test strips have not expired and have been stored in a closed container.
- Bilirubin
  - The dipstick detects conjugated bilirubin.
  - Unconjugated bilirubin is bound to albumin and does not pass through the glomerulus. Conjugated bilirubin however can pass freely through the glomerulus. The renal threshold for bilirubin is lower in the dog, especially male dogs, so low levels of bilirubinuria in that species is a common finding and is not considered an indication of disease. However, in cats, any amount of bilirubinuria is considered abnormal.

- A positive test indicates bilirubin overflow due to obstruction or cholestatic disease in the liver and hemolytic disease.
- Blood
  - Dipsticks are sensitive to free hemoglobin, intact erythrocytes and myoglobin. Hemoglobinuria is often reddish brown and clear and the color will not change with centrifugation. The plasma is also red in these patients. Myoglobinuria is more brownish; however, can look very similar to hemoglobinuria and also will not clear with centrifugation. The plasma in patients with myoglobinemia is not discolored. Hematuria consists of intact erythrocytes in the urine. The urine is red and will clear with centrifugation.
  - An ammonium sulfide test can be performed to distinguish myoglobin from hemoglobin. Add 2.8 g of ammonium sulfate to 5.0 mL of urine. If there is hemoglobin present, it will precipitate and myoglobin will not.
  - Causes of hematuria
    - Hematuria can occur secondary to any disease that injures the urogenital tract such as inflammation, neoplasia, or trauma including cystocentesis.
    - In addition, hematuria can be seen during the estrous cycle of some species.
  - Causes of hemoglobinuria
    - Severe hemoglobinuria can result from intravascular hemolysis. These patients are also anemic. Mild hemoglobinuria can occur with lysis of red blood cells in the bladder, especially if the patient has a low USG.
- Protein
  - The urinalysis dip stick is most sensitive to albumin.
  - Proteinuria can be a significant indication of disease. The kidneys should reliably filter protein, and therefore, the urine should be a very low protein fluid.
  - When interpreting the significance of proteinuria, it is very important to evaluate the USG and the urine sediment. If the patient has proteinuria with an inactive sediment and a low specific gravity, this is likely an indicator of kidney disease.
  - Concentrated urine can have low amounts of protein, also presence of enough blood to grossly discolor the urine or inflammation can result in elevated protein in the urine without renal disease. A thorough urinalysis is necessary to appropriately interpret the protein level.
  - Causes of proteinuria
    - Hemorrhage, including blood contamination from cystocentesis
    - Inflammation, often combined with hematuria
      - It is fairly common for a patient with cystitis to have mild to moderate proteinuria.
    - Renal disease
      - Both glomerular and tubular disease can result in significant proteinuria, often in dilute urine with inactive sediment. The proteinuria associated with glomerular disease (3+−4+) is often much more significant rather than tubular disease (1+−2+).
    - False positive tests can occur in alkaline urine, usually with a pH of 9 or greater or if there is peripheral blood contamination as can occur with cystocentesis. If the test strips are out of date, variable results can occur.

- Other tests are available to confirm the presence of proteinuria or more accurately quantify the protein.
  - Urine protein/creatinine (UPC) ratio
    - This test is used to evaluate the amount of protein excreted in urine while considering the patient's glomerular filtration rate or overall renal function. A healthy animal should have a UPC of <0.4. An abnormal ratio is a one-time value of >1 or repeatable values of >0.5. Patients with renal tubular disease often have values between 1 and 3 while patients with glomerular disease often have values >3.0.
  - Microalbuminuria
    - Urine dipsticks measure 30 mg/dL of protein or greater. Special testing is available which can measure smaller amounts of urine. The main test available is an ELISA and is available at many diagnostic laboratories.

Urine Sediment

A. Sample preparation
  - After the USG and urine chemistry are performed, the sample is ready to be centrifuged. A minimum of 5 mL of urine is necessary for accurate evaluation of the urine sediment. A well-mixed urine sample is placed in the centrifuge and spun for 5 minutes and 2000 rpm. The supernatant is poured off and the sediment is resuspended with a few drops of supernatant that remain in the tube. This can be done by flicking the bottom of the tube until the sample is well mixed. The poured off supernatant can be saved for additional testing such as UPC. One drop of sediment is placed on a glass slide and a coverslip is placed on the drop. The sample is now ready for microscopic evaluation. The sediment can be evaluated unstained or stained but an unstained sediment is ideal. Many of the available stains readily grow bacteria and form crystals that can be misleading when evaluating the sediment. All urine sediment images in this text are from unstained sediment preparations.
  - The sediment is initially scanned using a low power objective microscope lens (10×). The microscope condenser can be lowered to increase contrast within the sample. Many structures are quantified at low power and described per low power field (/lpf), for example: 1–2 casts/l pf. Then the sample is evaluated at high power using the 40× objective lens. The condenser can be raised at this magnification or can remain low. Many cells are quantified at this power and described per high power field or /hpf. Oil immersion is not recommended because this is a wet mount sample and if the objective touches the coverslip, the contents of the sediment disperse.
B. Contents of urine sediment
  - Cells in urine consist of epithelial cells, red blood cells (RBCs), and white blood cells (WBCs) or leukocytes.
    - There are three types of epithelial cells that can be identified in the urine sediment; squamous, transitional, and renal.
      - Squamous epithelial cells are not considered clinically significant. Squamous epithelial cells line the distal urethra and vagina and are commonly

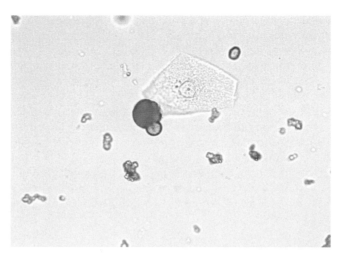

Figure 5.9   Urine sediment from a dog. Pictured is a single large angular squamous epithelial cell and many ammonium birurate crystals. The squamous epithelial cell has a small round nucleus with a moderate rim of cytoplasm. The borders are often at straight angles rather than round (50×).

observed in free catch and catheterized specimens. These cells are large and with abundant amounts of polygonal to irregularly shaped cytoplasm (Figure 5.9).

- Transitional epithelial cells line the renal pelvis, ureters, bladder, and proximal urethra. These cells can occur in urine from healthy animals in low numbers and are usually of no clinical significance. Samples obtained via catheterization can have high numbers of clusters of uniform epithelial cells. The only time that these cells are significant is if they are neoplastic. Transitional epithelial cells are round, smaller than squamous epithelial cells but larger than white blood cells. They have a moderate amount of cytoplasm with a centrally placed round nucleus (Figure 5.10). Patients with transitional cell carcinoma or bladder cancer can occasionally pass neoplastic cells in the urine. These cells are often large with large irregular nuclei and marked variability in cellular and nuclear size (Figure 5.11). If there is a suspicion that the cells could be neoplastic, a direct smear can be made of the sediment and that can be submitted for cytologic evaluation by a pathologist (Figure 5.12).
- Unlike squamous and transitional epithelial cells, renal epithelial cells are always significant and indicate underlying renal damage. These cells are smaller than transitional epithelial cells but slightly larger than white blood cells. They are round with a scant rim of cytoplasm and round, often a centrally placed nucleus (Figure 5.13). They may occur as individualized cells or as small cohesive cellular clusters.
- Red blood cells or erythrocytes are quantified per high power field of magnification (with the 40× objective lens). >4–5 cells/hpf is considered abnormal. Erythrocytes can be round or crenated depending on the USG. These cells are smaller than white blood cells (Figure 5.14a–c).

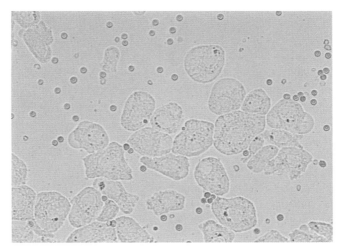

Figure 5.10   Urine sediment from a dog. The sample was obtained via placement of a urinary catheter so many transitional epithelial cells are observed. These cells are round with single round nuclei (50×).

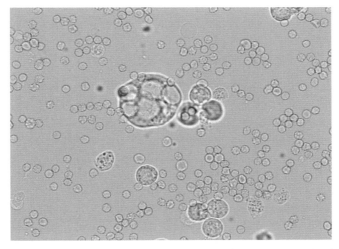

Figure 5.11   Urine from a dog with transitional cell carcinoma. Even in an unstained sediment smear the cellular atypia can be identified. Pictured is a large multinucleated cell. Red blood cells and few individualized transitional epithelial cells are present in the background (50×).

- Urine obtained via cystocentesis commonly has moderate numbers of red blood cells. The presence of red blood cells in the urine is termed hematuria.
- White blood cells are larger than red blood cells and they have a nucleus and many organelles and granules in their cytoplasm giving them a granular appearance (Figure 5.15a). White blood cells can occur in large aggregates or individually (Figure 5.15b). Normal urine from healthy animals can contain 3–5 cells/hpf. >5 WBCs/hpf is considered abnormal. Sometimes, so many

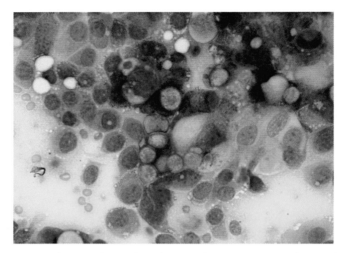

Figure 5.12   Direct smear of urine sediment from the same dog as Figure 5.11. The sample was stained with Wright–Giemsa. Clusters of atypical epithelial cells are identified exhibiting many criteria of malignancy including variation in cell size and nuclear size. The cells also contain eosinophilic mucinous material within the cytoplasm, typical for neoplastic transitional and prostatic epithelial cells (Wright–Giemsa stain, 50×).

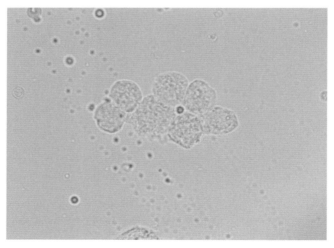

Figure 5.13   Urine from a horse. A cluster of renal tubular epithelial cells are present. The cells are small and round with a scant rim of cytoplasm. (100×).

white blood cells are present, the cells cannot be counted, and the sample is interpreted as TNTC or too numerous to count (Figure 5.16). In hypertonic urine, these cells can shrink and in hypotonic or alkaline urine, WBCs can lyse.
• The presence of increased numbers of WBCs in the urine is called pyuria.

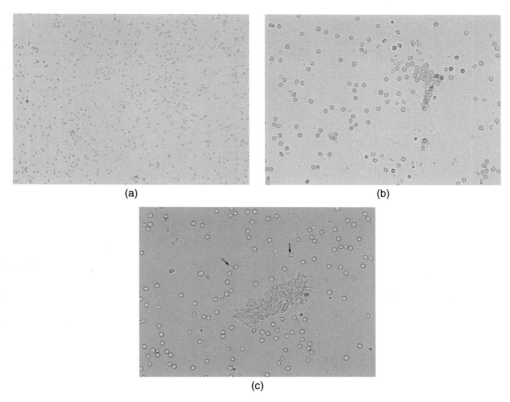

Figure 5.14   (a) Urine from a dog, the urine was collected by cystocentesis. Many red blood cells are identified (10×). (b) Same urine sample as (a). A higher power view allows for a more thorough evaluation of the cells. The red blood cells are small and anucleate. In dogs, the central pallor of the red blood cells is more obvious. (c) Urine from a dog with many red blood cells and a cluster of transitional epithelial cells. The arrows indicate red blood cells that are crenated. This is a common finding in urine. The indicated red blood cells have small cytoplasmic projections (50×).

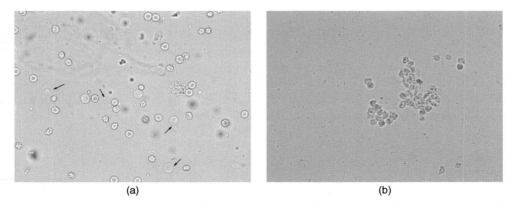

Figure 5.15   (a) Urine from a cat. White blood cells are indicated by arrows. Note that the white blood cells have a granular appearance and are larger than the red blood cells (50×). (b) Urine from a dog. Aggregates of white blood cells are identified admixed with many bacterial organisms. When the cells are in aggregates, they become more challenging to enumerate (40×).

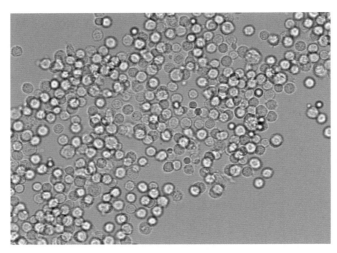

Figure 5.16   Urine from a cat. Full field of white blood cells are observed and may be described as too numerous to count or TNTC (50×).

TECHNICIAN TIP 5-3   Red blood cells can appear very similar to lipid droplets. Focus up and down on these structures with the microscope to differentiate these structures. Lipid droplets will be quite refractive when adjusting focus and red blood cells will just come in and out of focus.

- Casts
  - *Urinary casts* are imprints of the renal tubules and are formed as protein precipitates, cells, and cellular debris are shed from the renal tubules. The precipitated protein is a mucoprotein called Tamm-Horsfall mucoprotein. They can be considered normal in low numbers and are quantified /lpf. They are formed in the distal tubules and, when present in higher numbers (1 or more/lpf), they are considered indicative of renal damage, or primarily renal tubular disease. Casts are intermittently shed, therefore, they cannot be used to evaluate the severity of disease. The absence of casts does not eliminate renal disease as a cause of clinical disease. Casts form in acid urine and will dissolve in alkaline urine. These structures are tubular in shape with parallel walls (Figure 5.17). They are classified based on their internal structure and are described in the following list.
  - Epithelial casts
    - These structures consist of protein and sloughed renal tubular epithelial cells (Figure 5.18). They are commonly associated with toxic insults to the liver. Horses receiving gentamycin antibiotics are commonly evaluated for casts because these antibiotics are nephrotoxic.
  - Granular casts

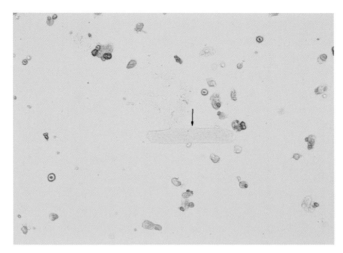

Figure 5.17   Urine from a dog. The arrow indicates a cast. The tubular structure has uniform and parallel walls (20×).

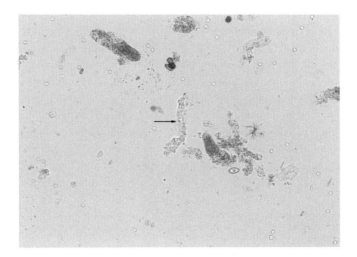

Figure 5.18   Urine from a horse. The arrow indicates a cellular cast, likely renal tubular cellular cast (50×).

- Often is the result of degeneration of cellular casts or cellular debris. Their internal structure varies from fine to coarsely granular (Figure 5.19a and b). Their presence in higher numbers indicates renal tubular damage.
- Waxy casts
  - These casts are considered a progression from granular casts. They are easy to recognize with little internal structure. They are thought to indicate chronicity of disease.
- White blood cell casts

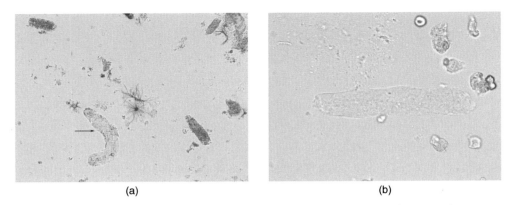

(a)   (b)

Figure 5.19   (a) Urine from a dog. The arrow indicates a combination coarsely and finely granular cast (20×). (b) Finely granular cast from the urine of a dog (50×).

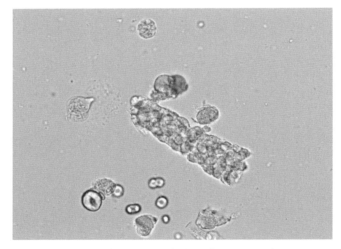

Figure 5.20   A single white blood cell cast is pictured. The cells are trapped in a proteinaceous material allowing them to maintain the tube-like structure in the urine. The presence of white blood cell casts indicates inflammation in the kidney (50×).

- Inflammation within the nephron will often result in the formation of these casts. They consist of white blood cells embedded in protein with the classic cast shape (Figure 5.20).
- Red blood cell casts
  - These occur with renal hemorrhage and are always considered pathologic. The casts appear brown to colorless and usually contains moderate numbers of red blood cells embedded in the protein matrix.
- Hyaline casts
  - These casts are 100% protein with no internal structure and are challenging to identify (Figure 5.21). Hyaline casts are usually considered

Figure 5.21   Hyaline cast in urine from a dog. These casts are 100% protein and can be very difficult to see in urine.

Figure 5.22   Urine from a cat containing many rod-shaped bacterial organisms and few white blood cells. Bacteria can be seen without staining the sample (50×).

nonpathogenic. They can occur in low numbers with anesthesia, fever, and exercise and in greater numbers in patients with glomerular disease.
- Microorganisms
  - Bacteria are the most common organisms identified in urine. Both cocci and rod-shaped bacteria can be identified (Figure 5.22). Cocci organisms are easiest to identify in chains, and individual cocci are often over-diagnosed and can be confused with cellular debris or contaminants (Figure 5.23). Urine is considered sterile until the midurethra so a cystocentesis is considered the best sample for culture.

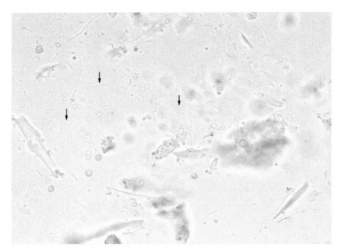

Figure 5.23   Urine from a dog containing much debris. This can make identification of bacteria challenging, and arrows indicate bacterial organisms (50×).

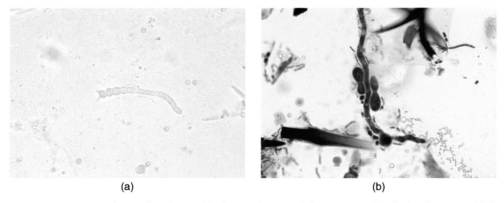

(a)   (b)

Figure 5.24   (a) Urine from a dog obtained by free catch. Fungal elements are identified and are most likely contaminant (100×). (b) Same urine as (a). A direct smear of the urine sediment was prepared and stained with Wright–Giemsa (100×).

- Fungal organisms are generally considered a contaminant, especially hyphae or chains of *Cyniclomyces guttularis*, which is a saprophytic yeast and normal flora of rabbit feces (Figure 5.24a and b).
- Occasionally systemic fungal infections such as *Blastomyces dermatitidis*, *Cryptococcus neoformans* and *Aspergillus* sp. can be identified in the urine (Figure 5.25a and b). These organisms are not considered contaminants in the urine.
- Parasites
  - Several different parasites have been identified in the urine. Eggs of *Capillaria plica* (the canine bladder worm) and *Dioctophyma renale* (canine

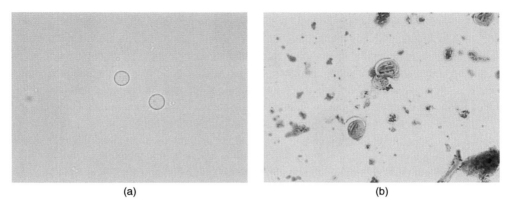

(a)   (b)

Figure 5.25   (a) Urine from a dog with systemic cryptococcocus. Few yeast organisms are present in the urine (100×). (b) Same urine from (a), a cytologic preparation of the urine sediment was stained with Wright–Giemsa. Low numbers of *Cryptococcus neoformans* yeast are observed (100×).

Figure 5.26   Urine sediment from a dog. A single *Pearsonema* sp. ovum was identified. Note the bilateral opercula (20×).

kidney worm) can be identified in urine sediment (Figure 5.26). Dogs infested with heartworm (*Dirofilaria immitis*) can occasionally shed microfilaria in the urine.

- Urine crystals form in fairly specific conditions. The urine pH can dictate which crystals will form and a change in the pH can lead to the dissolution of crystals. Older urine or urine with marked bactiuria may change pH after the sample is collected and if it is not evaluated fairly quickly, the crystals can dissolve. Temperature is also critical. Refrigeration can induce crystal formation and extreme heat can lead to crystal break down and result in a description of amorphous crystals in the urine. In addition, certain medications, particularly some antibiotics, can result in *crystalluria* (Figure 5.27).

Urinary crystals

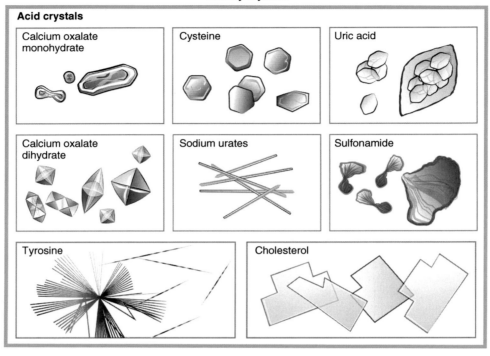

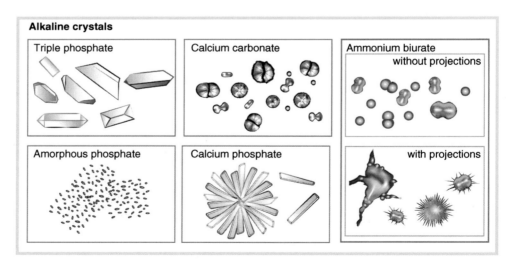

Figure 5.27   Examples of different crystal shapes.

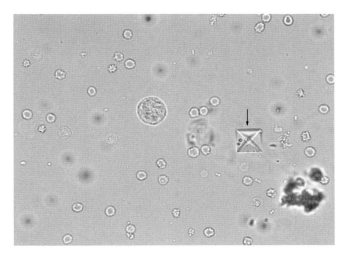

Figure 5.28   Urine from a cat. The arrow indicates a calcium oxalate dihydrate crystal, present in acidic urine. Also pictured are several red blood cells and a white blood cell (40×).

- Crystals found in acidic urine include calcium oxalate, cystine, hippuric acid, uric acid, and sulfonamide (Figure 5.28).
- Crystals formed in alkaline urine include triple phosphate (additional names for this crystal include struvite and magnesium ammonium phosphate), calcium carbonate, and ammonium biurate.
- Characteristics of individual urine crystals:
  - Ammonium biurate crystals can form in patients with liver disease or can be normal in certain breeds of dogs such as Dalmations. They are brownish gold in color and may be round and smooth (Figure 5.29) or have multiple thick projections (Figure 5.30).

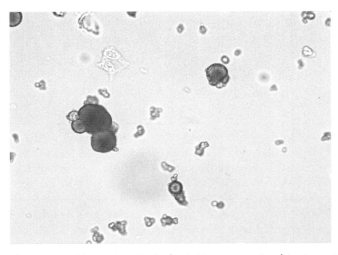

Figure 5.29   Urine from a dog with a portosystemic shunt. Many ammonium biurate crystals are observed. These crystals can be round with a typical brownish-gold staining (50×).

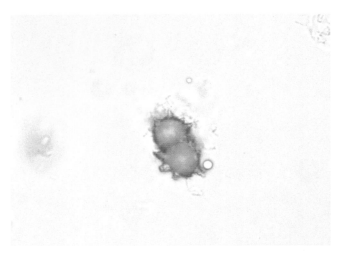

Figure 5.30   Urine from a dog with severe liver disease. Ammonium biurate crystals are also identified in this patient only these crystals have distinct projections (50×).

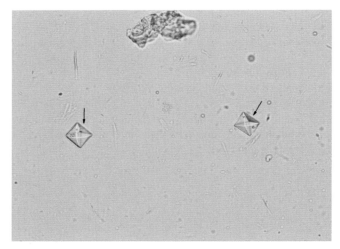

Figure 5.31   Urine from a dog. Arrows indicate calcium oxalate crystals are observed, they are square with a distinct x in the center (40×).

- Calcium oxalate dihydrate crystals can be seen in healthy dog and cat urine and are not necessarily an indication of disease unless the patient has evidence of stone (urolithiasis) formation. The most common shape of this crystal is square with an x in the center (Figure 5.31). These crystals can also appear more oval or diamond shaped (Figure 5.32).
- Calcium oxalate monohydrate crystals are not considered normal and are often associated with ethylene glycol toxicity or, in horses and cattle, may be associated with oxalate toxicity from plants such as rhubarb. Fortunately, these crystals look considerably different from calcium oxalate dihydrates.

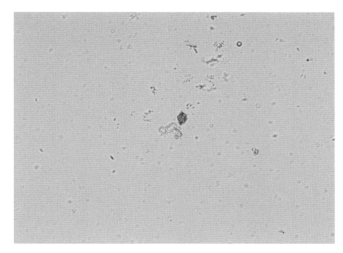

Figure 5.32   Urine from a dog. Calcium oxalate crystals can be variably shaped and the crystals pictured here are oval calcium oxalate dihydrate crystals (40×).

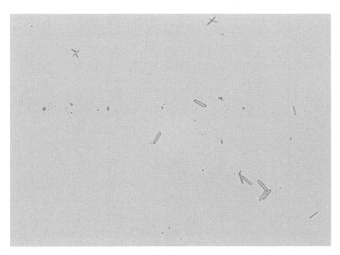

Figure 5.33   Urine from a dog that ingested ethylene glycol (antifreeze). Many calcium oxalate monohydrate crystals were identified. These crystals are often rectangular with a point at either end (50×).

They are rectangular with two sides coming to a point at both ends (Figure 5.33).

- Triple phosphate crystals can be seen in healthy dogs and cats and in dogs and cats with urolithiasis. Their shape resembles a coffin lid (Figure 5.34). They can dissolve very quickly if the urine acidifies.
- Cystine crystals are flat, six-sided crystals which are associated with an inherited defect in amino acid transport by the proximal renal tubule. Their presence is not really clinically significant; however, these animals are susceptible to urolith formation. Many dog breeds can be affected.

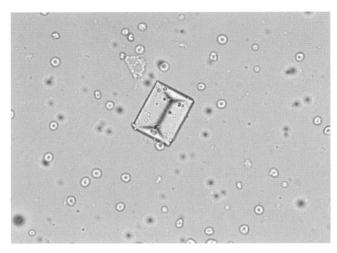

Figure 5.34   Urine from a cat with alkaline pH. A large triple phosphate crystal is imaged. Note the "coffin-lid" appearance of the rectangular crystal (50×).

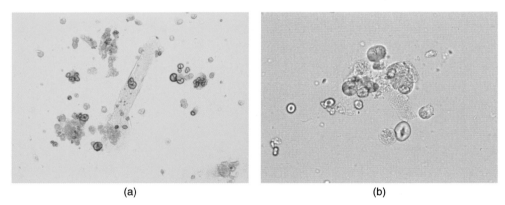

(a)   (b)

Figure 5.35   (a) Urine from a horse. Many calcium carbonate crystals are observed. These crystals are generally round with a golden-brown appearance (20×). (b) Urine from a horse. Calcium carbonate crystals that appear more oval are present but still have the characteristic golden-brown color (50×).

- Calcium carbonate crystals are considered normal in urine of horses and rabbits. They have many distinct shapes (Figure 5.35a and b).
- Bilirubin crystals can form in patients with bilirubinuria. These structures are brownish-gold aggregates of needle-like crystals that generally form in acidic urine (Figure 5.36).
- Urinary excretion of cholesterol crystals is uncommon in veterinary patients. They can be seen in diseases associated with severe tissue damage such as nephritis or pyelonephritis. The crystals are large and flat and are often notched.
- Several medications can induce crystal formation. Possible mechanisms include alteration of urine pH, alteration of glomerular filtration rate,

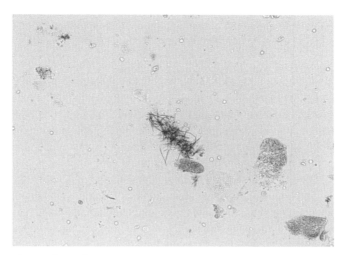

Figure 5.36   Urine from a dog with *Leptospira* sp. This patient had severe liver and kidney disease. In this image are filamentous bilirubin crystals. Casts were also noted in this dog's urine (50×).

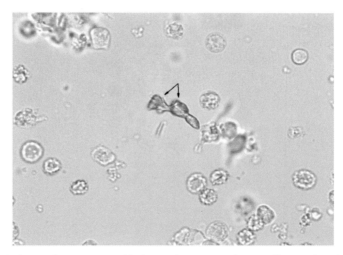

Figure 5.37   Urine from a dog receiving sulfa drugs. The arrows indicate sulfa crystals. White and red blood cells are also present (50×).

inhibition of tubular reabsorption, induction of tubular secretion, or precipitation of the drug in urine. Drugs implicated in crystal formation include sulfonamides (Figure 5.37), although newer generation sulfonamides are less of a problem, allopurinol used to treat Dalmations with uric acid uroliths and ampicillin.

- Amorphous crystals are often the result of dissolving crystals. As the crystals start to dissolve over time or the pH of the sample changes, the resulting crystals formed are amorphous.

- Miscellaneous structures
  - Lipid droplets are commonly identified, especially in canine and feline urine. These structures are round and can be difficult to differentiate from RBCs (Figure 5.38). Lipid droplets are refractile so if you focus up and down on them they will become very bright as they come in and go out of focus. RBCs will just appear blurry as they go out of focus.
  - Sperm are identified in intact male animals and are of no clinical significance (Figure 5.39). However, if there are many sperm in the urine, this can result in a mild increase in protein concentration.

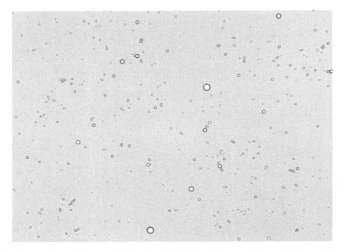

Figure 5.38   Urine from a dog. Many variably sized lipid droplets are observed. These structures are important to distinguish from red blood cells (50×).

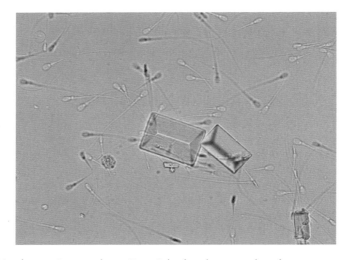

Figure 5.39   Urine from an intact male cat. Two triple phosphate crystals and many sperm are imaged (50×).

Figure 5.40   Urine from a dog. *Alternaria* sp. are considered an environmental contaminant. There distinct features should not be confused with a parasite ova or pathogenic fungus (50×).

- Pollen grains and other plant structures can appear similar to parasite eggs or fungal elements (Figure 5.40). Recognition of this material as a contaminant is critical.

Further Reading

Albasan, H, Lulich J.P., Osborne, C.A., *et al.* (2003) Effects of storage time and temperature on pH, specific gravity, and crystal formation in urine samples from dogs and cats. *Journal of the American Veterinary Medical Association*, 222(2), 176–179.

Bagley, R.S., Center, S.A., Lewis, R.M., *et al.* (1991) The effect of experimental cystitis and iatrogenic blood contamination on the urine protein/creatinine ratio in the dog. *Journal of Veterinary Internal Medicine*, 5(2), 66–70.

Ettinger, S.J. & Felman, E.C., (eds) (2010) *Textbook of Veterinary Internal Medicine!* (7th ed). St. Louis, MO: Saunders Elsevier.

Graff, L. (1982) *A Handbook of Routine Urinalysis*. Lippincott Co., Philadelphia, PA.

Hurley, K.J., & Vaden, S.L. (1998) Evaluation of urine protein content in dogs with pituitary-dependent hyperadrenocorticism. *Journal of the American Veterinary Medical Association*, 212(3), 369–373.

Latimer, K.S. (ed) (2011) *Duncan & Prasse's Veterinary Laboratory Medicine Clinical Pathology*, (5th edn). Wiley-Blackwell, Ames, IA.

Lyon, S.D., Sanderson, M.W., Vaden, S.L., *et al.* (2010) Comparison of urine dipstick, sulfosalicylic acid, urine protein-to-creatinine ratio, and species-specific ELISA methods for detection of albumin in urine samples of cats and dogs. *Journal of the American Veterinary Medical Association*, 236(8), 874–879.

Rees, C.A., & Boothe, D.M. (2004) Evaluation of the effect of cephalexin and Enrofloxacin on clinical laboratory measurements of urine glucose in dogs. *Journal of the American Veterinary Medical Association*, 224(9), 1455–1458.

Thrall, M.A., Weiser, G., Allison, R.W., & Campbell, T.W. (eds) (2012). *Veterinary Hematology and Clinical Chemistry*. Ames, IA: Wiley-Blackwell.

Vaden, S.L., Pressler, B.M., Lappin, M.R., *et al.* (2004) Effects of urinary tract inflammation and sample blood contamination on urine albumin and total protein concentration in canine urine samples. *Veterinary Clinical Pathology*, 33(1), 14–19.

Watson, A. (1998) Urine specific gravity in practice. *Australian Veterinary Journal*, 76(6), 392–398.

Whittemore, J.C., Gill, V.L., Jensen W.A., *et al.* (2006) Evaluation of the association between microalbuminuria and the urine albumin-creatinine ratio and systemic disease in dogs. *Journal of the American Veterinary Medical Association*, 229(6), 958–963.

Activities

Multiple Choice Questions

1. Turbid urine indicates:
   A) Highly concentrated urine
   B) An active sediment
   C) The sample was obtained by catheterization
   D) The urine pH is elevated

2. The glomerulus is responsible for:
   A) Filtration
   B) Resorption of glucose
   C) Resorption of water
   D) Production of hormones

3. Which technique is preferred for collection of urine for culture?
   A) Manual expression
   B) Free Catch
   C) Catheterization
   D) Cystocentesis

4. Which cell lines the bladder?
   A) Renal tubular epithelial cells
   B) Transitional epithelial cells
   C) Squamous epithelial cells
   D) All of the above

5. Increased white blood cells in the urine indicate:
   A) Hemorrhage
   B) Not significant
   C) Inflammation
   D) Trauma

6. Which is true of renal casts?
   A) They are formed in the distal renal tubule
   B) WBC casts can indicate inflammation in the tubule
   C) They are tubular in shape
   D) All of the above

7. Which crystal can be seen in urine from healthy horses?
   A) Calcium oxalate
   B) Calcium carbonate
   C) Ammonium biurate
   D) Triple phosphate

8. Which crystal forms in alkaline urine?
   A) Calcium oxalate
   B) Cystine
   C) Triple phosphate
   D) Uric acid

9. Ethylene glycol toxicity can result in the formation of this crystal:
   A) Triple phosphate
   B) Ammonium biurate
   C) Cystine
   D) Calcium oxalate monohydrate

Parasitology

chapter **6**

*Allan Paul[1], Amelia G. White[2] and
Anne M. Barger[1]*
[1]*University of Illinois, Champaign, IL, USA*
[2]*Auburn University, Auburn, AL, USA*

Learning Objectives

1. Understand the different techniques for fecal
   evaluation and the different applications.
2. Learn the different types of parasites.
3. Be able to recognize the morphology of
   parasite ova.
4. Be able to differentiate parasite ova from
   contaminants.
5. Understand the different testing for
   Dirofilaria immitis and the different
   applications.

KEY TERMS

Parasite
Protozoa
Round worm
Vector
Tapeworm
Hookworm
Whipworm
Fecal flotation
Passive flotation
Centrifugal fecal flotation
Sheather's solution
Baermann test

Clinical Pathology and Laboratory Techniques for Veterinary Technicians, First Edition.
Edited by Anne Barger and Amy MacNeill.
© 2015 John Wiley & Sons, Inc. Published 2015 by John Wiley & Sons, Inc.
Companion Website: www.wiley.com/go/barger/vettechclinpath

Case example 1

This is a fecal floatation from a dog with severe diarrhea. The large round eggs are consistent with round worms. Patients infected with round worms will sometimes pass adult worms in the vomit.

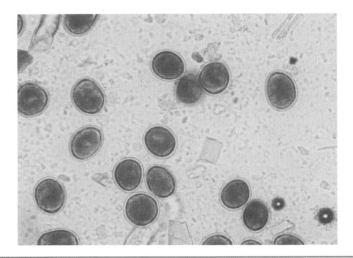

Case example 2

A mixed breed puppy presented with severe diarrhea, several weeks duration. A fecal floatation revealed low numbers of coccidial ova.

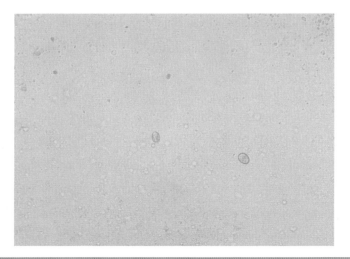

Introduction

Parasites are organisms that require a host to survive. Animals are exposed to many different parasites in the environment, from eating feces of other species, through mother's milk or placenta so it is very common especially for young animals to have a heavy parasite load. Diagnostic testing and appropriate therapy are critical for the health of the patient. Many of the parasites discussed in this chapter exist in the gastrointestinal (GI) tract; therefore, clinical signs for many of these parasites include diarrhea and vomiting. Parasites can also live on the skin and in the blood and these will be discussed to a lesser extent.

Classifications of Parasites

Many different classifications of parasites are described in the following list. It is important to understand the different classifications of the parasites because they all have different life cycles and respond to different therapeutics.

A. *Protozoa*: unicellular eukaryotic organisms. Include many groups with important parasites of animals and humans. Amoeba (Entamoeba), ciliates, flagellates (Trichomonas), and hemoflagellates (trypanosomes), Apicomplexa (e.g., the coccidians Eimeria and Toxoplasma, and the blood parasites – Babesia and malaria).
B. Platyhelminths: Flat worms
  • Trematoda: Flukes
    • Digenea – endoparasites with a complex life cycle that includes two or more hosts and environmental stages; many parasites of veterinary importance, such as the liver flukes and the lung flukes.
  • Cestoidea: *tapeworms*.
  • Cestoda – multisegmented worms, often with a complex life cycle and environmental stages; many parasites of veterinary importance, including beef tapeworms and Dipylidium in dogs and cats.
C. Nematoda: *round worms*
  A large group with many parasites of veterinary importance, including the strongyloids, hookworms, pinworms, and filarial worms; relatively little morphological heterogeneity, but vast differences in size and life cycles.
D. Arthropoda
  • Insecta – many parasites of veterinary importance.
  • Acari – ticks and mites include many parasites of veterinary importance.

Life Cycle

The host is the main environment for parasites (at least during one life stage). Parasites may be internal (endoparasites) or external (ectoparasites). A large number of parasites are intestinal parasites. The host GI tract is a unique environment, which offers several advantages to the parasitic life cycle. Some endoparasites are never found outside a host (e.g., protozoa and filarial nematodes that are *vector*-borne parasites).

A. Types of parasitic life cycles
  - Simple or Direct: only one host is required. Some parasites with a direct life cycle are transmitted directly from host to host (e.g., sexual transmission of *Trichomonas foetus* in cattle), while most pass through the environment (e.g., Giardia, Eimeria, and many nematodes).
  - Complex or Indirect: at least two hosts are involved. Parasites may or may not have contact with external environment during the life cycle. Examples include all digenean trematodes and many cestodes, which typically have one or more intermediate host, and vector-borne parasites, primarily protozoa and filarial nematodes (e.g., dog heartworm and human malaria), which are transmitted directly between vertebrate hosts and arthropod vectors.
B. Successful completion of the life depends on some or all of the following:
  - Host contact
  - Reaching an appropriate site in or on a host
  - Attachment and survival in/on the host
  - Feeding and reproduction
  - Exiting or releasing eggs or larvae out of the host
  - Survival in external environment
C. Modes of transmission
  - Free living stage ingested by host (passive)
  - Free living stage penetrates host (active)
  - Intermediate host ingested by definitive host
  - Vector transmission
  - Parasites can increase probability of transmission by modifying host behavior and through synchronization of their life cycle with the host life cycle.
  - Parasites can be acquired from soil, water, food, intermediate hosts, vectors, other animals, and one's self.
  - Common portals of entry utilized by parasites are skin, mouth, respiratory system, transplacental, transmammary, and sexual transmission.
    - Fecal-oral transmission through eating feces containing parasite eggs is a common way for new hosts to become infected by a parasite.

Effect of the Parasite on the Host

- Direct effects
  - Feeding and destruction of tissues
  - Production of toxins
  - Inhibition of host and host tissue or cell growth
- Indirect effects
  - Host allergic and hyperimmune responses

- Secondary infections
- Effect on competition and predation
- Often, the most deleterious effects may be found when a parasite is in the wrong host, or the wrong parasitic stage is in the host.

Endoparasites

Diagnostic testing

A. Fecal Evaluation
   - One of the most common laboratory procedures performed in veterinary practice is the fecal examination for the diagnosis of parasite infections. Fecal exams not only ensure the health of the animal but also help minimize the chance of transmission of potentially zoonotic parasites.
   - Fecal examinations can record the presence of parasites in multiple body systems. Parasites living in the GI tract produce cysts eggs or larvae that pass in the feces. Respiratory parasites produce eggs or larvae that are coughed up and swallowed and passed in the feces. Ectoparasites can also be found in feces as animals can swallow them when chewing or gnawing at their skin. Thus, it is important for the veterinary technician to have the knowledge and understanding of the multiple techniques utilized for fecal examinations.

> TECHNICIAN TIP 6–1   When collected from the environment, the fecal sample should be taken from the middle of the dropping to minimize contamination from environmental organisms.

   - Sample collection and storage
     - Samples should be as fresh as possible.
       - Either obtained rectally or dropped naturally.
         - Rectal collection can be performed with a fecal loop (Figure 6.1) or a gloved finger.
         - Several grams of fecal material are necessary to perform an adequate analysis.
         - Small amounts of feces such as found on a thermometer or even a fecal loop can produce false negatives because of small amount of feces and low numbers of eggs.
     - Samples should be refrigerated rather than frozen as soon as possible after collection. Freezing of the sample can damage organisms, making diagnosis much more challenging.
       - Store samples in airtight containers such as screw top jars (Figure 6.2) or baggies with air removed.

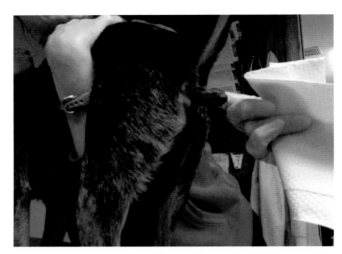

Figure 6.1   Fecal loops often do not collect enough feces to perform an adequate parasite examine. Manual removal of feces with a gloved hand will yield the appropriate volume of feces.

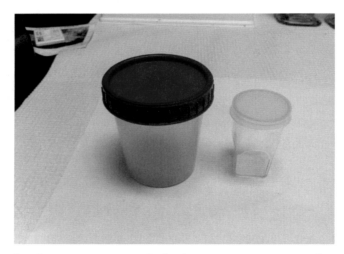

Figure 6.2   Examples of appropriate containers for fecal storage or transport. A complete and tight seal is important to keep the sample fresh.

- If the sample is submitted to a commercial or diagnostic laboratory, their protocols for preserving and shipping samples should be obtained before sending.
- Diagnostic tests
  - Direct smear
    - This test is used to identify motile protozoal organisms such as *Giardia* sp. and Trichomonads.
    - Technique

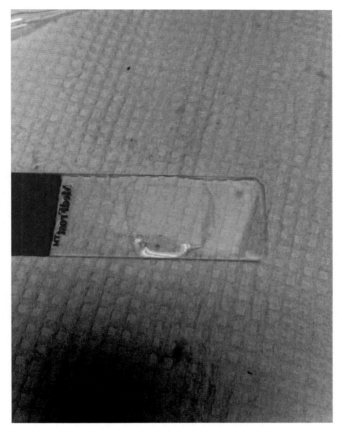

Figure 6.3   A small amount of feces is mixed with saline and covered with a coverslip is used to perform a fecal direct smear.

- A small amount of feces is mixed with a drop of saline on a microscope slide and covered with a coverslip (Figure 6.3).
- The sample should be evaluated first at 10× and then at 40×. Because this is a wet-mount preparation, oil immersion is not recommended because the structures of interest will move as the objective lens touches the coverslip.
- The layer of material should be thin enough to read newsprint.
- After examination, a drop of Lugol's iodine can be added to make the internal structures of the trophozoites easier to identify (Figure 6.4a and b).
- Fecal floatation
  - *Fecal flotation* is the most commonly used technique in veterinary practice for the examination of feces and identification of parasite ova.
  - The technique is based on the differences in specific gravity among the eggs, fecal debris, and the flotation solution. Parasite eggs present in the feces are less dense than the fluid solution and therefore should float to the top of the

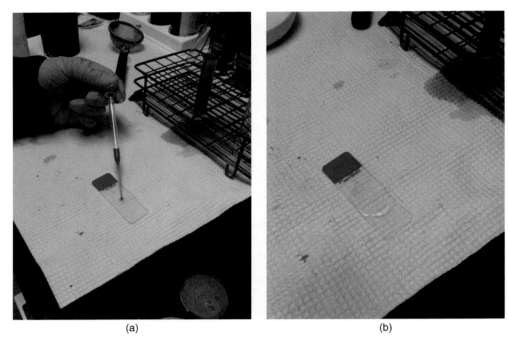

(a)   (b)

Figure 6.4   Lugol's Iodine can be added to a fecal direct to make structures easier to identify. (a) A drop is added to the saline and fecal mixture and (b) covered with a coverslip.

Table 6.1   Fecal testing solutions.

Flotation Solution	Specific Gravity
Fecasol (sodium nitrate)	1.2
33% Zinc sulfate solution	1.18
Saturated sodium chloride	1.2
Magnesium sulfate solution (Epsom salts)	1.32
Sheather's sugar solution	1.25

Solutions used for fecal testing and the specific gravity of each.

container. Solutions with a higher specific gravity are ideal because that will allow a greater variety of parasite ova to float to the top of the solution.

- Most parasite eggs have a specific gravity of 1.050–1.230; therefore, a solution with a specific gravity >1.2 works best for most parasites (Table 6.1). However, the greater the specific gravity of the solution is , the greater will be the risk of damaging the parasite ova.
- *Passive Fecal Flotation*
  - A common method used in clinical practice and is an important component of total animal health.

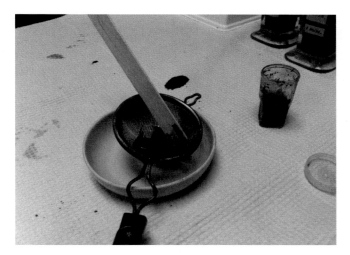

Figure 6.5   A small strainer can be used to remove large fecal material.

- This method relies on gravity to separate parasites and debris.
- This test is easy to perform; however, because many of the common flotation solutions are similar in specific gravity to some parasites, this technique can result in false negatives. The centrifugation technique is a more sensitive technique.
- Zinc sulfate or saturated salt solutions can be used for standard fecal flotation.
- Several grams of feces are mixed with the solution and strained through a tea strainer or cheesecloth (Figure 6.5).
- The mixture is then poured into a test tube until a reverse meniscus is formed and a coverslip is added to the top (Figure 6.6a and b).
- The solution should stand for 15 minutes and then the coverslip is removed, placed on a microscope slide, and examined (Figure 6.7).

TECHNICIAN TIP 6–2   If a fecal flotation sample sits too long, the solution can begin to crystallize making evaluation difficult.

- Centrifugal fecal flotation
  - This is the preferred technique and gold standard for fecal flotation.
  - *Sheather's sugar solution* is commonly used for this technique; however, 33% zinc sulfide flotation solution can also be used.
  - This method has been shown to recover significantly more eggs and has fewer false negative results than passive flotation systems.
  - Necessary supplies
    - Swinging bucket centrifuge
    - Porcelain bowl or other fecal container

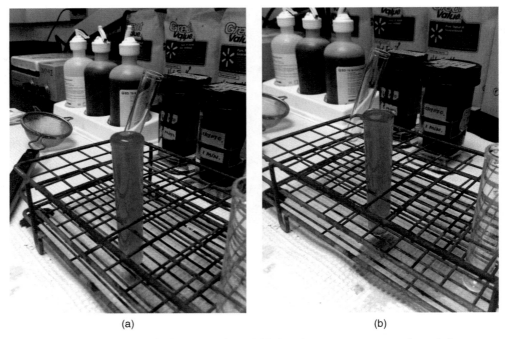

(a)   (b)

Figure 6.6   (a) The mixture is added to a test tube and filled until a reverse meniscus is formed. (b) A coverslip is then placed on top.

- Strainer
- Tongue depressor
- 15-mL plastic centrifuge tube
- Technique
  - Mix 5–10 grams of feces with 15 mL of water in the porcelain bowl.
  - Strain the mixture
  - Use a tongue depressor to mix the feces in the strainer, breaking up any clumps and mashing well.
  - When well mixed, lift the strainer from the bowl. Examine the contents of the strainer for worms or larvae. If none are visible, discard the contents in a biohazard container and rinse and clean the strainer.
  - Use a tongue depressor to stir the liquid contents of the bowl to resuspend any parasite ova. Fill a 15-mL plastic centrifuge tube within $1/2$ inch from the top.
  - Place the tube in a swinging bucket centrifuge making sure that it is appropriately counterbalanced.
  - Centrifuge the sample for 5 minutes at 1500–1750 rpm. Allow the centrifuge to stop on its own.
  - Discard the supernatant without disrupting the pellet. Add Sheather's sugar solution within $1/2$ inch from the top. Resuspend the pellet and supernatant.

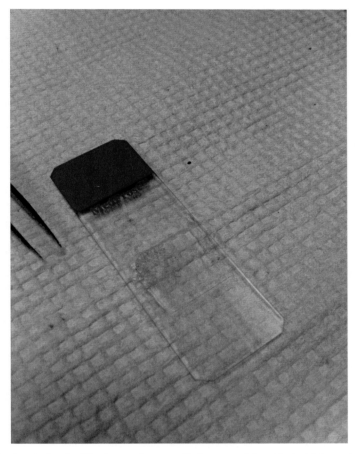

Figure 6.7   After incubating for 15 minutes, the coverslip is removed from the test tube and placed on a microscope slide for systematic microscopic evaluation.

- Place the tube back in the centrifuge and add enough Sheather's sugar solution to form a positive meniscus. Place a coverslip on top of the tube and gently press down to seat it on top of the tube. Counterbalance the tube in the centrifuge.
- Centrifuge the sample for 10 minutes at 750–800 rpm. If the coverslip comes off during the spin, then this step should be repeated after more Sheather's solution is added and a new coverslip is placed.
- After the centrifugation has been completed (let the centrifuge stop on its own without applying the brake) remove the coverslip by lifting it straight up and place it onto a microscope slide for examination.
- Examine the entire slide using a back and forth pattern to ensure completeness.
- Thoroughly clean the centrifuge before the next use.

> **TECHNICIAN TIP 6–3**   If using a centrifuge with an angled rotor (the tubes are not straight up and down when the sample is not spinning) fill the tube as high as possible and centrifuge the sample without a coverslip on top. When the centrifugation is complete, remove the tube and place it in a rack and fill the tube with solution and then place a coverslip on top. Let that sample sit for an additional 15 minutes. Then remove the coverslip and examine microscopically.

- Microscopic examination of slides
  - Slides should be examined on low power (10×).
  - Examine the whole area under the coverslip. Start at one corner of the slide and scan the slide up and then down in several rows to ensure thorough examination of the whole area.
  - If there is question to the identity of the structure, closer examination at 20× or 40× is possible. Oil immersion is challenging with wet-mount slides such as fecal samples because the objective comes in contact with the coverslip and often material within the sample will move in response to the contact.
  - If the slide has an unusual parasite or structure that requires consultation with a veterinary parasitologist, paint the perimeter of the coverslip with nail polish. This will seal in the liquid and limit the amount of air that can cause the sample to dry up. The slide can then be shipped to a diagnostic laboratory or university for further review.
- Quantitative fecal examinations
  - There are several quantitative fecal techniques. Two of the more commonly used are the McMaster's quantitative test and the Wisconsin quantitative test.
  - Egg counting techniques are used primarily in horses. These techniques are used to estimate the extent of parasite egg contamination for growing animals on pastures or to determine whether drug-resistant parasites are present. Fecal egg counts can be useful in developing herd deworming programs.
  - Egg counts, however, are not a reliable way to diagnose parasitic disease in individual animals. Many factors can affect egg production including species of worm present, individual immunity, and stage of infection. Egg counts for individual animals are best interpreted when combined with other factors such as clinical signs, history, and Faffa Malan chart (FAMACHA) score.
- McMaster's quantitative test
  - Using a balance, weigh out 2 grams of fecal material. Place into a tea strainer resting in a porcelain bowl.
  - Add 28 mL of half-strength sheather's sugar solution to the bowl (14 mL sheather's solution and 14 mL tap water).
  - Once well mixed, lift strainer, press excess liquid out of the solids, and collect it in the same bowl. Discard the solids.
  - Stir the liquid in the bowl to resuspend and immediately pipette up the solution.

- Fill both chambers of a McMaster's counting slide.
- Let it sit undisturbed for at least 20 minutes before continuing.
- Count separately, each egg type or oocyst found under the gridded areas of both sides of the counting slide. (i.e., count ascarids separate from trichostrongyles, separate from coccidian, etc.)
- Multiply each tally by 50 to obtain an answer in eggs/gram of feces.
- Wisconsin quantitative test
  - Procedure
    - Combine 5 grams of feces and 20 mL of water in a plastic container and mix into a slurry.
    - Pipet 1 mL of the slurry to a centrifuge tube used for passive floatation.
    - Fill the tube with Sheather's solution to a mild inverse meniscus.
    - Place a coverslip on the tube and centrifuge for 10 minutes at 750 rpm.
    - Remove the coverslip and place on a glass slide. The slide should be evaluated systematically using the 10× objective lens of a microscope.
    - Separately count each egg type or oocyst found under the entire surface of the cover slip.
    - Divide each tally by five to obtain an answer in eggs per gram of feces.
- Baermann test
  - The *Baermann technique* is used to recover larvae from the feces of animals with lung or intestinal parasitic infestations where the diagnostic stage is a larvae rather than an egg. The test is based on the movement of the larvae out of the feces and into warm water so they can be collected and identified. It is very important that fresh fecal samples be used as free living nematodes or larvae hatched from eggs can make proper identification difficult with time.
  - Technique
    - The Baermann technique can be performed using a variety of methods but the basic setup can be seen in Figure 6.8.
    - The setup is as follows:
      - One end of a piece of latex tubing is attached to a funnel and a clamp is placed on the other end.
      - The funnel is placed in a ring stand.
      - The fecal sample is wrapped in cheesecloth and placed on a piece of wire mesh.
      - The sample is placed into the funnel and the setup is filled with warm water.
      - The sample is left in the funnel for 12–18 hours.
      - Slowly release the clamp and let the first 10 mL of the sample drain into a conical test tube (Figure 6.9).
      - Centrifuge the test tube at 1500–1750 rpms for 5 minutes. Discard the supernatant and examine the sediment on a microscope slide for larvae.
- Fecal Sedimentation
  - The sedimentation technique is used primarily to identify eggs of flukes and some tapeworms that do not float well in common flotation solutions due

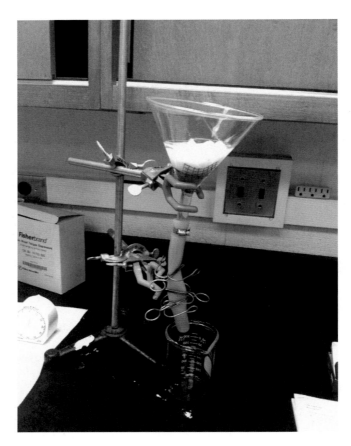

Figure 6.8   Pictured is the basic Baermann apparatus.

to high specific gravity or the presence of operculum. This technique allows
for eggs and debris to settle at the bottom of a container.

- Technique
  - Break up the fecal sample in a 1% liquid soap solution in a 50-mL
    conical tube and then fill the tube to the top with the soap solution.
  - Let the sample stand undisturbed for 5–10 minutes, then carefully decant
    or aspirate off the supernatant, being cautious to lose none of the
    sediment.
  - Refill the tube with the 1% soap solution and repeat the procedure three
    to five more times until the supernatant is relatively clear.
  - Examine the sediment on a microscope slide for the presence of fluke
    eggs, which are usually large, clear amber eggs with an operculum.
  - Adding one drop of 0.1% methylene blue will stain the background
    debris but will not stain fluke eggs thus allowing the amber colored eggs
    to stand out.

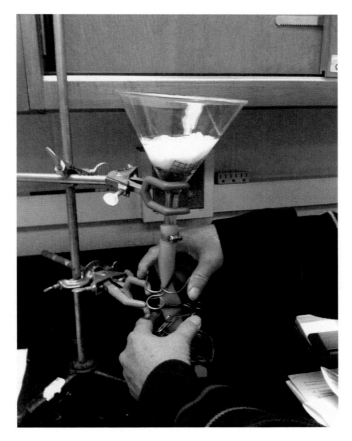

Figure 6.9   The clamps of the apparatus are released and the first 10 mL are collected.

- Fecal cytology
  - Patients that present with diarrhea can have a fecal swab or rectal scrape performed. This diagnostic test is used to evaluate microorganisms in the feces such as bacteria, fungal organisms and occasionally protozoa or ova. The rectal scrape is generally performed by a veterinarian; however, fecal cytology smear can easily performed in a laboratory setting.
- Fecal smear
  - This technique can be performed easily from a fecal sample obtained for fecal flotation. A cotton-tipped applicator is placed in the feces and then smeared on a slide.
  - The slide is allowed to air-dry and then can be stained with Romanowski type stains such as Diff-Quik®.
  - The slide is then examined microscopically. Bacteria are the primary organisms to be examined so microscopic evaluation at 100× with immersion oil is beneficial. If evaluation is performed at 40×, place a coverslip on the slide to increase the quality of the image. A mixed

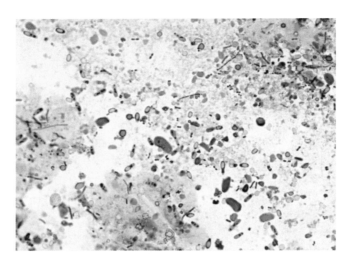

Figure 6.10   Fecal smear from a dog with diarrhea. Multiple clostrideal organisms are observed (100×).

population of bacteria will be identified in feces from healthy animals but there are organisms that are recognized as known pathogens such as *Campylobacter* sp. and *Clostridium* sp. Low numbers of clostridial organisms can be identified in feces from healthy animals but if there are multiple organisms/100× field, there is a concern for clostridial overgrowth, especially if the patient has diarrhea. Morphologically, these organisms are rod shaped with a single spore either at one end of the organism (resembling a tennis racket) or in the middle (resembling a paperclip) (Figure 6.10). *Campylobacter* sp. organisms should not be present in feces from healthy animals so even low numbers of these organisms are considered pathogenic. They are curved, similar to a comma and can form chains, which allow them to appear similar to spirochetes or spiral shaped bacteria (Figure 6.11). Fungal yeast organisms can also be identified in fecal smears and are often considered overgrowth or contaminants. Few fungal organisms including *Blastomyces dermatitidis*, *Histoplasma capsulatum*, and *Cryptococcus neoformans* have been reported in feces and are considered true (Figure 12) pathogens (Figures 6.12–6.14). In addition, a saprophytic yeast, *Cyniclomyces* sp., which is considered normal flora of the rabbit GI tract, can also be observed in canine feces. It is unclear if these organisms are pathogenic in dogs.

B. Heartworm testing
- Dogs and cats are at risk of heartworm infestation (*D. immitis*). The adult worm lives in the right heart and pulmonary arteries. It is a deadly disease in both dogs and cats. *Dirofilaria immitis* is transmitted by mosquito bite. Adult worms in the dog produce microfilaria. The microfilaria circulates in the blood. The mosquito bites an infected dog and ingests the microfilaria. The larvae of *D. immitis* matures in the mosquito and when it reaches the third stage, it migrates to the

Figure 6.11   Fecal smear from a dog with diarrhea. Many *Campylobacter* sp. organisms are observed in chains giving them the appearance of a spirochete (100×).

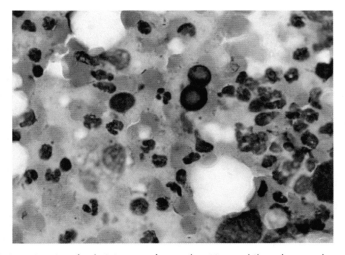

Figure 6.12   This is an imprint of a draining tract from a dog. Neutrophils and macrophages are observed with a budding fungal yeast organism consistent with *Blastomyces dermatitidis* (100×).

mosquito's salivary gland. When the mosquito bites a dog, the third stage larvae enters the bite wound where it matures to a fourth stage larvae. Within 2–3 months after inoculation, the fourth stage larvae mature to a young adult and migrate to the pulmonary artery where it starts producing micorfilaria. This can take 6–9 months after infection. The adult worms can grow to be 3.2–11 cm in length.

- Accurate testing and prevention is a vital component the canine and feline patient health.

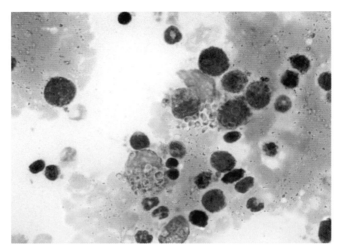

Figure 6.13   Rectal scrape from a dog. Inflammatory cells including macrophages, neutrophils, and small lymphocytes are present. *Histoplasma capsulatum* yeast is identified in the cytoplasm of the macrophage and free in the background (100×).

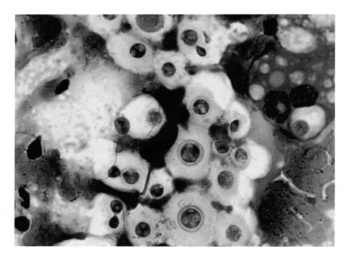

Figure 6.14   Intestinal lymph node aspirate from a dog with diarrhea. Many fungal yeast organisms consistent with Cryptococcus neoformans are identified. Note the narrow based budding and nonstaining capsul (100×).

- Diagnostic testing in dogs can involve identification of the adult worms or microfilaria.
  - Adult worms
    - Antigen testing
      - Worms must reach the adult stage before an antigen test is positive. This usually occurs 6.5 months after infection and the detection of antigen can

occur before identification of microfilaria. For this reason, there is no reason to test puppies less than 6 months of age.

- The manufacturer's instructions should be followed exactly otherwise results may be unreliable or misleading.
- Weak positive tests should be confirmed with another test method such as testing for microfilaria. If false positive tests occur, it is usually due to poor technique, especially inadequate washing of the sample.
- False negative tests can occur. The antigen is specific to female worms so if the patient has too few mature female worms, a negative test is possible.
- Retesting of dogs on an annual basis is important especially in patients that live in an area where the risk of exposure is high, if growth beyond the weight range of the initial dose of preventative was calculated, or if compliance of administration of preventative is uncertain.

- Demonstration of microfilaremia
  - These tests are not as sensitive and specific as testing for the antigen directly
  - Direct blood evaluation
    - A drop of blood is placed on a slide and covered with a coverslip. The sample is evaluated for movement of the microfilaria (Figure 6.15). May not be able to detect with low numbers of circulating microfiliaria.
    - Two types of microfilaria can be seen *D. immitis* (heartworm) and *Acanthocheilonema reconditum* formerly *Dipetalonema reconditum*. These organisms can be difficult to differentiate (Table 6.2).
    - Occasionally, microfilariae can be identified on a blood smear prepared for a CBC.
  - Microhematocrit tube examination
    - Technique
      - Draw whole blood into microhematocrit tube.

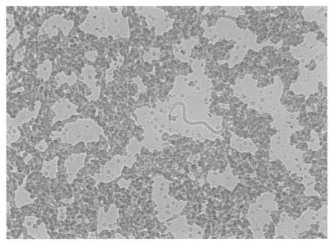

Figure 6.15   Wet mount of blood for evaluation for microfilaria. A microfilaria is identified as well as many red blood cells (20×).

Table 6.2   Data used to differentiate *Dirofilaria immitis* from *Acanthocheilonema reconditum*.

	Dirofilaria immitis	*Acanthocheilonema reconditum*
Relative number of microfilaria	Usually many	Few
Motion in direct smear	Coiling and flexing	Coiling and progressive movement across field

Size
    1. Length
    2. Width
	286–340 μ
	6.0–7.4 μ
		246–294 μ
		4.3–5.8 μ

Body shape	Straight	Curved
Tail shape	Straight	Buttonhook or straight
Head shape	Tapered	Blunt
Cephalic hook	Not present	Present

Comparison morphological data *for Dirofilaria immitis* and *Acanthocheilonema reconditum*.

- Centrifuge for 5 minutes in a microhematocrit centrifuge.
- Microscopically examine the area where the buffy coat contacts the plasma using the 10× objective lens.
- Microfilaria can be seen moving just above the buffy coat.
- May not detect low numbers of microfilaria, not a sensitive assay.
- Species differentiation is not possible with this technique.
- Modified Knott's test
  - Technique
    - Add 1 mL of either freshly drawn blood, blood in ethylenediaminetetraacetic acid (EDTA), or blood with heparin to 10 mL of 2% formalin in a 15-mL, plastic conical bottom centrifuge tube.
    - Mix the sample by gently pipetting.
    - Let sit 2–5 minutes to allow the formalin to lyse the red blood cells.
    - Centrifuge for 5 minutes at 1500 rpm.
    - Pour off the supernatant and dispose of appropriately. About 1/2 mL of solution will remain in the tube; this is normal.
    - To the remaining fluid add 4–7 drops of 1/1000 methylene blue. Mix by gently pipetting. Let stand 2–5 minutes to allow sediment to resettle.
    - Pipette two or three drops of the sediment from the bottom of the tube and apply to a microscope slide. Place a coverslip on the material and examine microscopically for microfilariae.
- Heartworm disease in cats is considerably different than in dogs. Infected dogs can have dozens of adult worms in their pulmonary artery. Cats rarely have more than a few adult worms. In addition, cats do not have microfilaria in circulation. Cats develop severe respiratory disease as young adult worms migrate through

the lungs. In addition, heartworms in cats can migrate to locations other than the cardiovascular system and cats can die suddenly from the disease.
- Diagnostic testing in cats is considerably different than in dogs. Antigen tests are often negative because of the low number of adult worms in cats.
  - Antibody testing
    - Measurement of heartworm antibodies suggests exposure to the parasite but not necessarily an active infection. Exposure of the patient to the larvae from an infected mosquito can result in production of the antibodies
    - This test is used most frequently in cats because they often have a low parasite burden with mature worms and therefore will likely not have enough antigens in circulation, which will result in false negative test results.
    - A snap test is available. The manufacturer's instructions should be followed closely.
C. Parasite Identification
  - Fecal parasites
    - Gastrointestinal parasites
      - Cestodes
        - Tapeworms are the most common cestode. Most species of domestic animals are at risk.
        - Dogs and cats can have two different families of tapeworms, *Dipylidium caninum* and *Taenia* spp.
          - In general, the adult tapeworms cause minimal problems. In large numbers, diarrhea and weight loss can occur. Proglottids may cause pruritis.
          - Often, the eggs of the organisms are not present in the feces but the proglottids can be identified in the stool. The proglottid of *D. caninum* resembles a cucumber seed and *Taenia* sp. resemble rice grains (Figure 6.16).
          - The intermediate host of *D. caninum* is the flea so dogs and cats infested with fleas are often at risk for tapeworms. To become infected with the tapeworm, patients must ingest the flea.
          - *Taenia* sp. is often acquired by ingestion of infected rodents.
      - Cattle
        - *Moniezia* spp. are a cestodes or tapeworms of cattle. The cattle get infested by ingesting the intermediate host, pasture mites, which contain the larvae. The adult tapeworms cause few if any problems.
        - Tapeworm segments can be seen in the feces but the eggs can also be seen in fecal flotations.
      - Horses and donkeys
        - *Anoplocephala* spp. and *Paranocephala mamillana* are tapeworms of equids. Owing to its location near the ileo-cecal valve, *Anoplocephala* spp. can cause colic due to obstruction of this valve. Other equine tapeworms cause few if any problems.
        - Fecal flotation for eggs is an insensitive test; however, antibody testing *Anoplocephala* spp. is available.

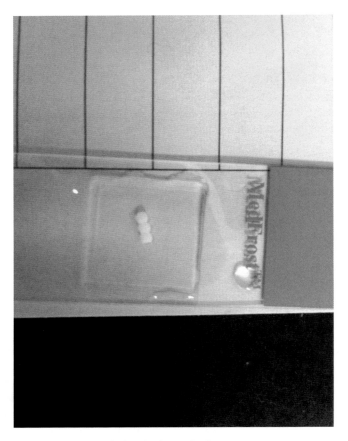

Figure 6.16   *Taenia* sp. segments identified in the feces of a dog.

- Nematodes
  - Dogs and cats
    - *Hookworms* are a fairly common parasite in puppies and kittens. The adult worm attaches itself or "hooks" onto the mucosa of the small intestine.
    - Animals become infected with hookworms most commonly from ingestion from the environment. In dogs, transmammary transmission can also occur; therefore, the puppies can become infected by nursing. Transmammary infection does not occur in cats.
    - Hookworms are voracious blood suckers. They leave anticoagulant at their feeding sites and the sites continue to bleed after they leave. The worms feed at 5–7 sites a day. Severe anemia, dehydration, and black tarry stools (melena) can be seen.
    - Organisms identified in dogs and cats are *Ancylostoma* spp. (common) and *Uncinaria stenocephala* (uncommon). Eggs can be identified in a fecal flotation (Figure 6.17).

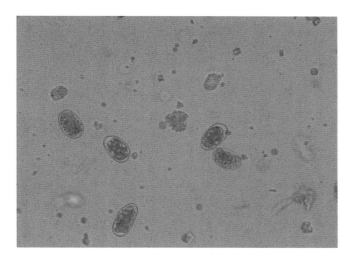

Figure 6.17   Passive fecal floatation from a dog. Many hookworm ova are identified (20×).

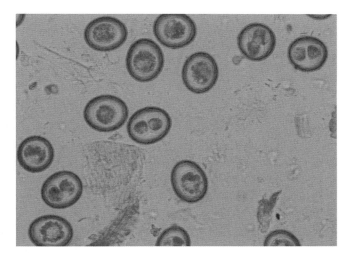

Figure 6.18   Fecal floatation from a cat. Many roundworm eggs (*Toxocara cati*) are identified (20×).

- *Roundworms* or *Toxocara* spp. are very common parasites. In dogs, transmission is by transplacental, transmammary or by ingestion of eggs in the environment. In cats, transmission is transport hosts and transmammary. Eggs are easily identified by fecal flotation (Figure 6.18).
- Roundworms can cause a variety of clinical signs including diarrhea and/or constipation, vomiting, weight loss, and dehydration. If there are large numbers of worms or a very heavy parasite load, intestinal obstruction can occur. Environmental control is also very important because people can become infected by ingesting eggs in the soil.

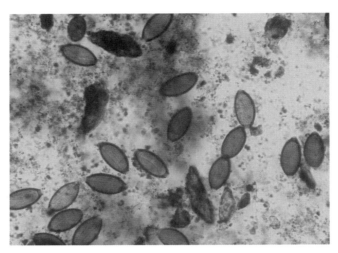

Figure 6.19   Fecal floatation from a dog. Many whipworm eggs are identified. Note the bilateral opercula (20×).

Toddlers are at the highest risk because they are not known for having a discriminating appetite. Soil commonly exposed to canine feces such as parks can be high risk for infection. Pet owners should be encouraged to clean up after their pets, especially in public areas.

- *Whipworms* are commonly diagnosed in dogs with only rare reports in cats. The canine whipworm or *Trichuris vulpis* is transmitted to dogs by ingesting infective eggs from the environment. Centrifugal flotation is a superior method for identifying ova. The ova have a unique appearance (Figure 6.19).
- Whipworms migrate in and out of the mucosa of the cecum and large intestine causing large amounts of damage. They feed off the blood and often produce a bloody diarrhea.
- Ruminants (Cattle)
  - Strongylid parasites include multiple genera of organisms including *Ostertagia* spp., *Haemonchus* spp., *Trichostrongylus* spp., and *Oesophagostomum* spp., to name a few. Transmission is by ingestion of larvae from the pasture. Most ruminants are infested with strongylid parasites. The ova can be identified in fecal flotation and are similar in morphology to the canine hookworm (Figure 6.20). The ova can appear very similar and often are described as "strongylid type" ova.
  - The parasites damage the intestinal mucosa, ingest blood, and can cause severe anemia. This is especially true in goats. Production losses are also a major concern.
  - Whipworms (*Trichuris* spp.) live in the cecum and colon of ruminants. The eggs look similar to those in the dog (Figure 6.21).
  - Hookworms in ruminants are similar to dogs, they ingest blood, damage the intestinal mucosa, and can cause severe anemia and bloody diarrhea.

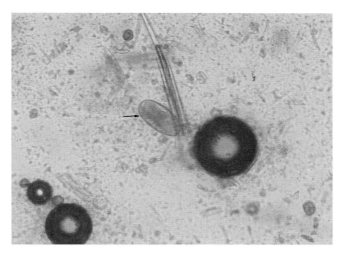

Figure 6.20   Fecal floatation from a cow. A strongyle egg (arrow) is identified. These organisms are very similar to the canine hookworm (20×).

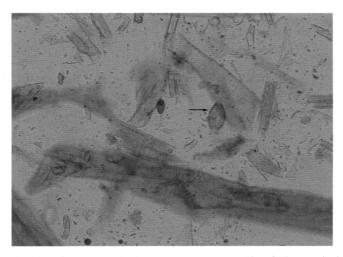

Figure 6.21   Fecal floatation from a cow. A whipworm egg (arrow) is identified. Note the bilateral opercula (20×).

- Nematodirus, also known as the thread-necked worm, are fairly common. The ova are quite large (Figure 6.22) and the organism rarely results in clinical disease within the patient.
- The most common roundworm identified in ruminants is *Toxocara vitulorum*. It can be readily identified in standard fecal flotation techniques. The nematode lives in the small intestine and can cause severe diarrhea in calves.

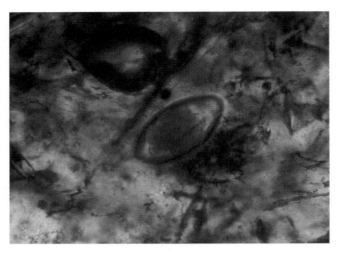

Figure 6.22   Fecal floatation from a cow. A large nematodirus ova is noted. These organisms rarely cause clinical disease (20×).

- Horses
  - Strongylid parasites are very common. The eggs resemble the canine hookworm. They live in the ceum and colon of infected horses and horses become infected from ingesting larvae from pastures.
  - *Parascaris equorum* is the equine roundworm. The adult parasite lives in the small intestine of horses and larvated eggs are ingested in infested pastures. Standard fecal flotation is adequate for diagnosis.
  - *Oxyuris equi*, or the equine pinworm, is of minimal clinical significance. Adult female worms from the adult horse deposit eggs near the perianal region where they potentially can be ingested. Clinically, these parasites may cause anal irritation but other clinical disease is not noted.
- Protozoa
  - Dogs and cats
    - Several species of coccidia (*Isospora* spp.) can be found in dogs and cats. Puppies and kittens can have severe diarrhea. Diagnosis can be made by passive or centrifugal fecal flotation. The ova are small and have distinct morphology (Figure 6.23).
    - *Toxoplasma gondii* oocysts are only seen in cats. It is transmitted by ingesting cysts from intermediate hosts. Oocysts can be identified in feces by both passive flotation and centrifugal flotation.
    - Giardiasis is a fairly common cause of diarrhea in dogs and less so in cats. Cysts are ingested in the environment. Identification of feces for cysts and to lesser extent trophozoites are possible. Trophozoites can be seen in direct saline smear or on fecal smears (Figure 6.24).

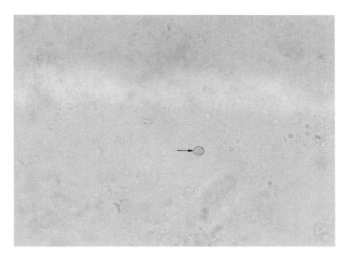

Figure 6.23   Fecal floatation from a dog. A small coccida ova (arrow) is identified (20×).

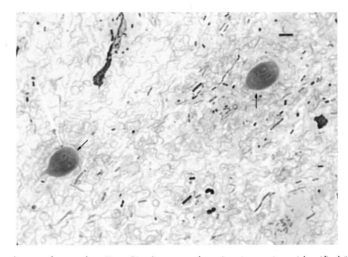

Figure 6.24   Fecal smear from a dog. Two *Giardia* sp. trophozoites (arrows) are identified (Wright-Giemsa, 100×).

- Ruminants
  - Coccidiosis in ruminants is commonly caused by *Eimeria* spp. Animals are infected by ingestion of oocysts from the environment. The organisms are easily recognizable with fecal flotation (Figure 6.25).
  - *Cryptosporidium* spp. is a common GI parasite in cattle and can result in severe diarrhea, particularly in calves. Centrifugal fecal flotation with Sheather's sugar solution or acid-fast staining should be used to identify the oocysts (Figure 6.26).
  - Ruminants are susceptible to *Giardia* spp. similar to dogs and cats.

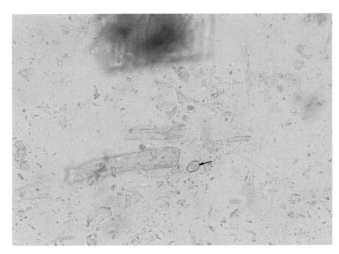

Figure 6.25   Fecal floatation from a cow. The arrow identifies a single coccidia ova. These ova are small and oval (20×).

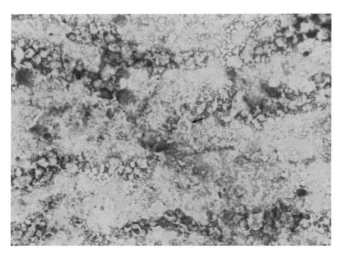

Figure 6.26   Acid-fast stain of feces from a calf with severe diarrhea. The arrow identifies a Cryptosporidial oocyst (50×).

- Equine
  - *Eimeria leuckarti* is the causative agent of coccidiosis in horses. Horses are infected by ingesting oocysts from the environment. Sedimentation or flotation can be used to identify the oocysts.
  - *Giardia intestinalis* and *Cryptosporidium* spp. can be diagnosed in horses similar to other species.
- Cardiopulmonary parasites
  - Nematodes
    - Dogs and cats

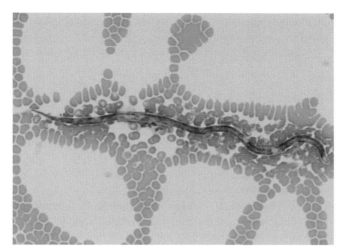

Figure 6.27   Blood smear from a dog. A microfilaria is present and should be confirmed as *Dirofilaria immitis* with a heartworm antigen test (Wright-Giemsa, 50×).

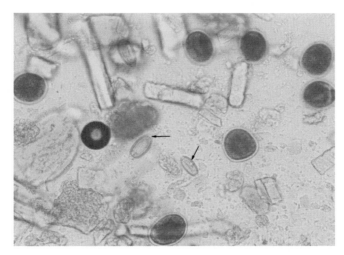

Figure 6.28   Fecal floatation from a cat. Many roundworm ova are identified; however, the arrows indicate *Capillaria aerophilus*. Similar to whipworms, these ova have bipolar opercula (20×).

- *Dirofilaria immitis* or heartworm is the most common cardiovascular parasite in dogs and cats. Microfilaria can be identified in peripheral blood and has distinct morphological features (Figure 6.27).
- *Eucoleus aerophilus* is a lung worm of dogs and cats, previously known as *Capillaria aerophilus*. The adult worm can be found in the trachea, bronchi, and bronchioles. The ova are identified via fecal flotation (Figure 6.28) or in fluid collected during a transtracheal wash (TTW) or bronchoalveolar lavage (BAL).

- *Aleurostrongylus abstrusus* is a lung worm found in cats. The patient often presents for coughing and may have a peripheral eosinophilia. The adult worm can be found in the lung parenchyma. Larva can be identified via TTW or BAL. First stage larva can also be identified in the feces, the Baermann technique is recommended.
  - Ruminants and horses
    - *Dictyocaulus* spp. or common lung worm can occur in cattle, sheep, goats, and horses. The adult worm lives in the trachea, bronchi, and bronchioles. The Baermann technique can be used to identify larva.
  - Trematodes
    - Dogs and cats
      - *Paragonimus kellicoti* can be found in the lung of dogs and cats as well as goats. The eggs can be identified in the feces with the sedimentation technique or in TTWs or BALs (Figure 6.29).
- Structures mistaken as parasites
  - Environmental fungus
    - *Alternaria* spp. is a conidia commonly found in the environment (Figure 6.30). The structures can also be seen in urine sediments.
    - Other fungal spores or hyphal structures can also be identified in feces and can resemble parasite ova.
  - Plant structures
    - Plant fibers can appear similar to fungal hyphae or other pathogenic structures but are common contaminants in fecal samples (Figure 6.31).
    - Pollen granules can be uniform and round with distinct walls and commonly are confused with parasite ova (Figure 6.32).

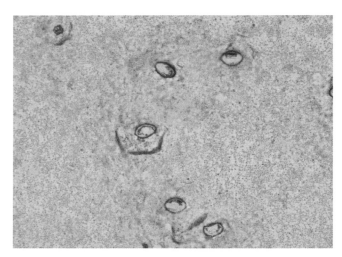

Figure 6.29   Transtracheal wash from a cat. Many large *Paragonimus kellicoti* ova are noted in a background of eosinophils and neutrophils (Wright-Giemsa stain, 10×).

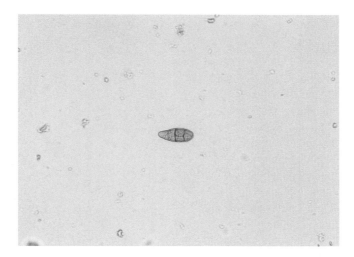

Figure 6.30   *Alternaria* sp. is merely common environmental contaminants (50×).

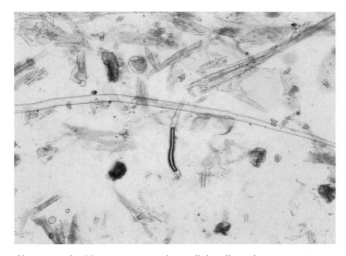

Figure 6.31   Plant fibers are tube-like structures with parallel walls and are contaminants and not parasites (20×).

- Nonpathogenic parasites
  - Grain mite eggs can commonly be observed in canine and feline feces. These organisms can be seen in feces from ingesting mite-infested food (Figure 6.33).
  - *Monocystis lumbrici* is a parasite of earthworms. If the earthworms are ingested, the spore can be identified (Figure 6.34).

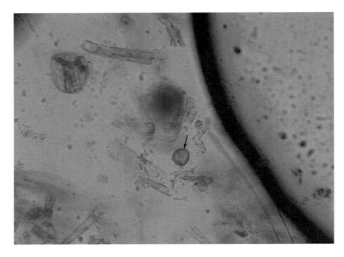

Figure 6.32   Pollen grains are common contaminants. There spiky surface (arrow) is unique (20×).

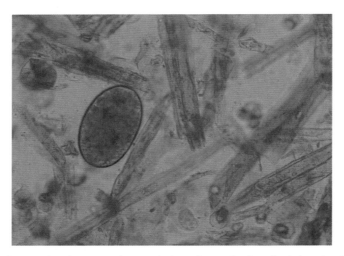

Figure 6.33   The large grain mite egg can be seen in feces from animals eating infested grain and is not a pathogenic parasite (20×).

Ectoparasites

These parasites are similar to endoparasites in that they require a host to survive; however, they are located on the outside of the host's body. These parasites gain their nutrients by consuming host materials such as blood, skin cells, and sebum or other skin by-products. Some of these parasites live completely on the outside of the host within the haircoat, such as fleas, ticks, and lice. Others burrow within the superficial layers of the skin or deeper within the epidermis such as *Sarcoptes* spp. and *Demodex* spp. mites. There are thousands of ectoparasites that can infest the skin of veterinary

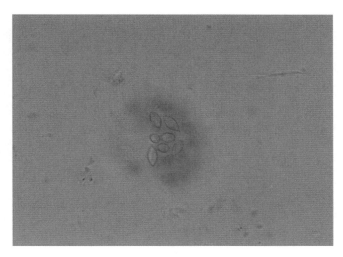

Figure 6.34   Ova from *Monocystis lumbrici*, the earthworm parasite, is not a parasite in mammals (20×).

patients, so only the most commonly observed parasites will be discussed in further detail.

Diagnostic testing

A. Cytology
   - Cytology can be useful when identifying mites located superficially on the surface of the skin.
   - Techniques (Figure 6.35)
     - Clear acetate tape is used in order to facilitate appropriate passage of light through the sample and transparency for microscopic evaluation. Do not use frosted tape. The sticky adhesive allows for better sampling and capturing of the parasites and eggs from the patient. This technique is best used for capturing large superficial ectoparasites.
       - Technique
         - Firmly press a 1-inch piece of clean, clear acetate tape directly to the skin repeatedly over lesional skin or visualized parasites.
         - Firmly adhere the tape to the glass slide and then examine it microscopically under low light intensity, low power (10×), and a closed condenser.
         - Note: an additional technique of squeezing the skin repeatedly with the tape attached has been shown to be useful for the detection of demodex mites in dogs. Examination of the tape is performed as described previously.
     - Direct impression smear – a glass slide can be pressed directly onto the lesional skin; however, this method is usually not rewarding for the collection of parasites from the skin, especially those that move quickly away from the slide but can be useful for other cytological analysis.

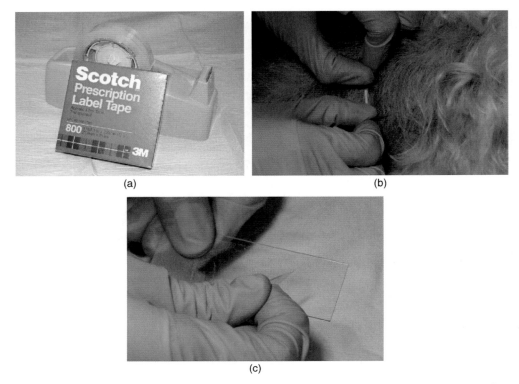

Figure 6.35   Clear acetate tape (a) is pressed firmly over the skin to collect a skin/hair sample (b), as well as any surface parasites. The tape is placed on a slide (c) and then observed under the microscope at low power.

- Fine needle aspirate – this technique can be used for evaluation of nodular or mass-like skin lesions; however, this method is usually not rewarding for examination of parasites in the skin but much more useful in diagnosis of inflammatory or neoplastic processes.
B. Skin scraping (Figure 6.36)
  - This technique is especially helpful for identification of lice and burrowing mites. Scrapings can be performed in a superficial or deep manner depending on the parasite of interest.
    - Superficial skin scrapings – this technique is used to identify parasites located in the superficial layers of the epidermis such as *Sarcoptes* spp. or *Notoedres* sp.
      - Technique
        - A small amount of mineral oil is applied to a clean glass slide. A clean number 10 scalpel blade is dipped into the mineral oil, or the mineral oil can be applied directly to the skin at the site of the skin scraping.
        - Holding the blade perpendicular to the skin or slightly deviated away from the direction of scraping, the blade is gently passed over large areas of the skin in a sweeping pattern.

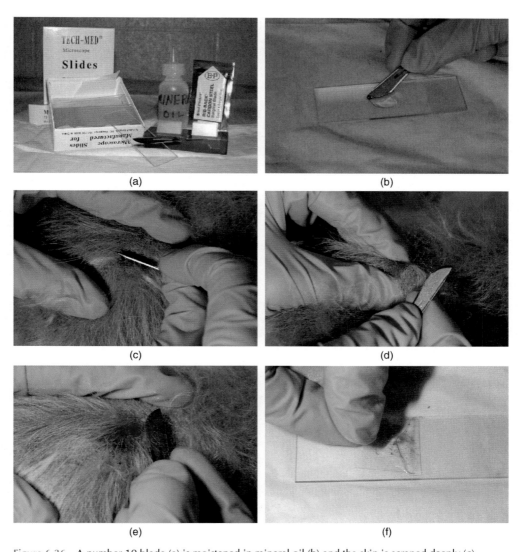

Figure 6.36   A number 10 blade (a) is moistened in mineral oil (b) and the skin is scraped deeply (c), periodically squeezing the skin between the thumb and forefinger (d), until blood is obtained (e). This material is put onto a glass slide in a small amount of mineral oil, a glass coverslip applied (f), and the slide observed under the microscope for parasites at low power.

- Skin material is collected within the mineral oil and placed on the glass slide. A glass coverslip is applied to the slide.
- The slide is examined at low power (10×), low light intensity, and a closed condenser for evidence of parasites (adults, larva, nymphs, and eggs).
- Deep skin scrapings – this technique is used to identify parasites located in the deeper layers of the epidermis such as *Demodex* spp. mites.
  - Technique

- A small amount of mineral oil is applied to a clean glass slide. A clean number 10 scalpel blade is dipped into the mineral oil, or the mineral oil can be applied directly to the skin at the site of the skin scraping.
- Holding the blade perpendicular to the skin or slightly deviated away from the direction of scraping, the blade is gently passed over a small area of lesional skin in a sweeping pattern. The skin should be pinched firmly between the thumb and forefinger to help extrude the parasites from within the deeper epidermal layers periodically when scraping. Scraping is performed until a mild amount of blood is seen grossly on the glass slide.
- Skin material and blood is collected within the mineral oil and placed on the glass slide. A glass coverslip is applied to the slide.
- The slide is examined at low power (10×), low light intensity, and a closed condenser for evidence of parasites (adults, larva, nymphs, and eggs).

C. Trichogram (Figure 6.37)
- This technique can be used to examine for evidence of parasites or eggs attached to hair shafts or for the presence of adult parasites deep in the hair follicle epithelium.
    - Technique
        - Using hemostats, tufts of hairs from lesional skin are rapidly removed from the animal. The sample is placed in a small amount of mineral oil on a clean glass slide, and a glass coverslip is applied to the slide.
        - The slide is examined at low power (10×), low light intensity, and a closed condenser for evidence of parasites (adults, larva, nymphs, and eggs). Eggs frequently are seen attached to hair shafts. Adult parasites may be seen at the base of the hair follicle, in the remaining follicular epithelium, or free floating within the mineral oil.

D. Fecal evaluation
- Parasites may be observed in the feces of animals when they are consumed during grooming. This occurs more commonly with ectoparasites that cause pruritus (itching).
- Evaluation is the same as previously described for endoparasites.

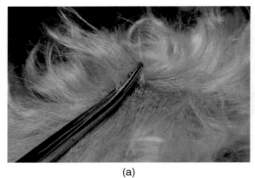
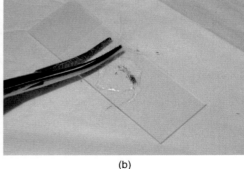

(a)   (b)

Figure 6.37   (a and b) When performing a trichogram, a pair of hemostats can be used to firmly grasp and remove hair from the patient. The hairs are placed in mineral oil on a glass slide, a coverslip applied, and the slide observed under the microscope for parasites at low power.

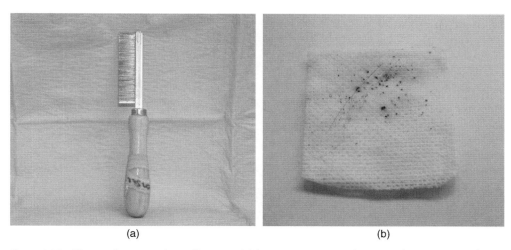

(a)   (b)

Figure 6.38   Flea combs are used to collect material from a patient (a), and a piece of wet gauze can be used to observe feces of fleas. Feces will cause a reddish-brown color when smeared onto wet gauze (b).

E. Combing and wet paper towel test (Figure 6.38)
   • Use of a flea comb or fine-toothed comb to collect skin, scale, parasites, eggs, and excrement can be useful to identify large ectoparasites.
      • Technique
         • A fine-toothed comb is passed repeatedly over the animal's entire body. It should be passed especially in locations where the ectoparasites are known to reside (i.e., the dorsocaudal tail base for fleas). Collected material can be examined grossly for parasite identification or microscopically if magnification is required.
         • In addition, any brown-colored debris consistent with parasite excrement of blood-sucking parasites can be confirmed as digested blood meals via use of the wet paper towel test. In this test, any material containing blood should smear or streak out with a red-brown coloration when using a wet paper towel or damp gauze.
F. Biopsy and histopathology
   • Because ectoparasites are so readily identified using the techniques described above, more invasive techniques, such as biopsy, are rarely required for identification of ectoparasites. However, this technique may be required when an intense inflammatory reaction occurs as a secondary response to the presence of the parasite. Depending on the size of the lesion, punch biopsy or excisional biopsy may be required for lesion removal. The specimen is immediately placed in 10% formalin until submitted for histopathological evaluation. This technique may not be as sensitive as those described previously.

Parasite Identification

Visualizing images of the parasites will be helpful when determining the parasite you are encountering in the clinical setting. This text does not include many images of ectoparasites. The authors encourage the readers to refer to other texts for images of ectoparasites including *Georgis' Parasitology for Veterinarians*, *Muller & Kirk's Small Animal Dermatology*, and *Veterinary Clinical Parasitology*.

A. Arachnids
  - Parasites belonging to the class Arachnida differ from insects because of the absence of wings, the presence of four pairs of legs in adults, and fusion of the head and thorax. Parasites belonging to this class include ticks, mites, and spiders.
    - Ticks
      - Ticks are blood-sucking parasites that belong to the suborder Metastigmata. They are classified into two major families: the Argasidae (soft) ticks and the Ixodidae (hard) ticks. Soft ticks are considered more primitive and less parasitic while hard ticks are much more specialized and highly parasitic.
      - Life stages
        - Ticks have four general life stages: egg, larva, nymph, and adult. Eggs are laid in several batches of hundreds for argasids and in a single clutch of thousands for ixodids. Larva hatch out of eggs, take a blood meal, and molt into a nymph. Many soft ticks molt through several nymphal stages before becoming an adult while hard ticks typically have one nymphal stage.
        - Hard ticks are classified as one-, two-, or three-host ticks. One-host ticks complete all molts on one host; however, nymphs drop off to molt in two-host ticks, and nymphs and larvae drop off to molt in three-host ticks.
        - Ticks attach to the host via a mouthpart composed of three structures: the hypostome with backward projecting teeth, the chelicerae that protects the hypostome, and the palps that move laterally while the tick is feeding. The hypostome is the main component that adheres the tick to the host while feeding. In addition, some ticks may produce a cement-like material for further stabilization during feeding. Argasid nymphs and adults feed repeatedly on the host while ixodids feed only once.
        - Hard ticks have a scutum, or shield, that covers the entire dorsal surface of the male and part of the dorsal surface of the female. This can aid in identification of the tick species. This scutum grows to accommodate the blood volume ingested. This is different from the cuticle of the soft tick that expands to accommodate the blood volume ingested.
      - Disease transmission
        - Ticks not only can cause anemia in the host when present in large numbers on one host or when a host has a relatively small blood volume (i.e., neonatal animals) but also transmit infectious diseases including bacteria, rickettsiae, protozoa, and viruses. Specific diseases will be discussed with each tick.
        - Owing to their long mouthparts, ticks can create painful bite wounds with significant secondary inflammation and infection.

- Ticks secrete harmful toxins from their salivary glands when feeding that can lead to tick paralysis.
- Family Argasidae (soft tick)
  - These ticks live in nests and burrows where they can attach to and feed quickly (minutes or hours only) on hosts. They prefer warmer environments and typically hide during the day and feed at night. While they usually parasitize birds, they can also infest all types of wild and domestic animals.
  - There are about 140 species of soft ticks that belong to four genera: *Argas, Ornithodoros, Otobius,* and *Antricola.*
  - Examples include the following:
    - Spinous ear tick: *Otobius megnini*
      - This is the only soft tick considered to be of significant concern to dogs and cats. It affects animals living in the southern and western United States. The larvae and nymph are found in the external ear canal where they commonly lead to otitis externa characterized by secondary bacterial/fungal infections, pain, and even convulsions. Other clinical signs include head shaking or scratching. Some animals may have asymptomatic infections.
      - The adult ticks are not considered parasitic and can live up to 6–12 months. Larvae can live unfed for 2–4 months and eat lymph produced by the ear. They are yellow to pink in color, 0.3-cm spherical ticks with three pairs of small legs. Larvae molt into bluish-gray nymphs with four pairs of legs within 5–10 days of feeding. Nymphs feed on host ear lymph for 1–7 months before molting into adults.
      - Treatment includes physical removal of ticks from ear canal, application of mineral oil to smother remaining ticks and use of insecticides such as pyrethroids to kills the ticks. Long-acting spot-on preparations with efficacy against ticks are recommended for animals at risk for reinfestation. Treating the environment is also important for prevention of reinfestation.
- Family Ixodidae (hard tick)
  - These ticks live in fields or other areas where they attach onto a passing host and feed for several days. Many of genera of hard ticks have been identified in the United States with several of them being responsible for the transmission of infectious diseases. We will briefly touch on some of the most common hard ticks in veterinary patients. Refer to other texts for a more thorough list of ticks and for more specific features of each tick especially as pertains to tick identification.
    - *Ixodes* spp.
      - An identifying feature of this tick is that the anal groove forms an arch anterior to the anus. Species of this tick commonly transmit infectious diseases such as Lyme disease, babesiosis, and ehrlichiosis in many animals and humans. This tick may also cause tick

paralysis. Common species in these genera include the deer tick, *Ixodes dammini*, and the black-legged tick, *Ixodes* scapularis.

- *Rhipicephalus* spp.
  - One of the identifying features of this tick is that the basis capituli is hexagonal in shape. Species of this tick commonly transmit infectious diseases such as babesiosis, anaplasmosis, ehrlichiosis, tularemia, and cause tick paralysis in many animals and humans. One of the most common species in these genera is *Rhipicephalus sanguineus*.
- *Dermacentor* spp.
  - An identifying feature of this tick is the basis capituli is rectangular shaped when viewed from above. Species of this tick commonly transmit infectious diseases such as Rocky Mountain spotted fever, tularemia, Colorado tick fever, Q fever, tick paralysis, babesiosis, and cause tick paralysis in many animals and humans. Common species of this tick include *Dermacentor variabilis* (brown dog tick), *Dermacentor andersoni* (Rocky Mountain wood tick), and *Dermacentor occidentalis* (Pacific or West Coast tick).
- *Amblyomma* spp.
  - Identifying features of this tick are mouthparts that are longer than the basis capituli and a longer second palpal segment. Species of this tick commonly transmit infectious diseases such as Rocky Mountain spotted fever, ehrlichiosis, tularemia, and cause tick paralysis. Common species of this tick include *Amblyomma maculatum* (Lone Star tick), *Amblyomma americanum*, *Amblyomma cajennense*, and *Amblyomma imitator*.
- Mites
  - These differ from ticks because they lack a leathery cuticle, the hypostome may lack supporting structures, and some have spiracles on the cephalothorax. The life cycle is similar among the members and include egg, larva, nymph, and adult.
- Superficial mites – these mites live within the hair, on the skin surface, or within the stratum corneum of the epidermis.
- *Sarcoptes* spp. (Figure 6.39)
  - This mite belongs to the family Sarcoptidae.
  - *Sarcoptes scabiei* causes sarcoptic mange or "scabies" in humans, dogs, foxes, horses, cattle, pigs, and other animals. There is considerable host specificity despite the wide range of animals affected (e.g., *Sarcoptes scabiei* var. *canis* causes disease dogs, cats, and foxes only). Scabies is reportable in cattle. *Sarcoptes scabiei* var. *canis* has been reported to live for up to 6 days on a human host.
  - This mite has a round to oval body (200–400 µm) with long, unsegmented pedicels (component of the pretarsi) ending with a suckers on the two pairs of anterior legs. The two posterior legs do not end in suckers, except for the last pair of legs in the male. The anus is located at the posterior edge of the body.

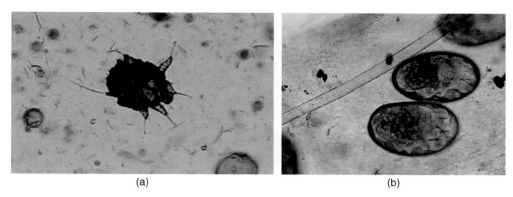

(a)   (b)

Figure 6.39   *Sarcoptes* sp. adult mite (a) and eggs (b) as observed under the microscope at low power (10×) from a superficial skin scraping.

- The life cycle is about 17–21 days. Adults live on the skin surface and burrow 2–3 mm/day into the stratum corneum to lay eggs. Larvae hatch from the eggs and molt into nymph and eventually adults within molting packets at the skin surface. Mites can survive for 2–6 days off of the host.
- *Sarcoptes* spp. live on the hairless areas of the body but may become generalized to all areas of the skin with chronicity. Typical areas affected on the dog include the lateral aspects of the pinna and legs and the ventrum.
- Clinical signs include alopecia, pruritus, papules, excoriations, and lichenification. Secondary infections are common. The disease is highly contagious by direct contact with and infected individual or through fomites (e.g., bedding).
- *Notoedres* sp.
  - This mite belongs to the family Sarcoptidae, and it causes feline scabies.
  - This mite typically affects cats (i.e., *Notoedres cati*), but it may cause disease in foxes, dogs, and rabbits. This mite is not common in all parts of the United States. *Notoedres douglasi* has been reported in two fox squirrels.
  - See *Sarcoptes* spp. for life cycle and description of mite. Differences are that the anus is located dorsally in *Notoedres* sp. mites, and the pedicels of the front legs are only medium length.
  - It is also considered highly contagious by direct contact with an infected animal or indirectly through fomites.
  - It typically affects the medial proximal edge of the ear pinna initially spreading rapidly to the upper ear, face, eyelids, and neck. It may even spread distally to the feet and perineum.
  - Clinical signs are the same as for scabies.
- *Chorioptes* spp.
  - This mite belongs to the family Psoroptidae.
  - This mite affects cattle primarily (*Chorioptes bovis*) but may also be found on the tail and legs of horses, sheep, and goats and the ear canal of rabbits.
  - The mite is round, 0.3–0.5 mm in length with short, unsegmented pedicels on the first, second, and fourth pairs of legs of the female and all legs of the

male. The mite resides superficially on the skin of the tail, rump, perineum, caudomedial thighs, caudal udder, scrotum, legs, and feet of cattle. It sometimes is referred to as "foot mange" or "tail mange." It can also be found in the ears of rabbits and on the body of hedgehogs. Transmission occurs by direct and indirect contact, and clinical signs are typically worse in the winter months.

- Clinical signs include erythema, pruritus, papules, crusts, excoriations, alopecia, restlessness, leg stomping, tail swishing/rubbing, and in severe cases weight loss, hide damage, and loss of production. Marked epidermal hyperplasia can occur with chronicity. In rams, it is associated with exudative dermatitis of the lower legs and scrota and decreased semen quality.

- *Psoroptes* spp.
  - This mite belongs to the family Psoroptidae.
  - The mite affects numerous animals including cattle (*Psoroptes bovis*), sheep (*Psoroptes ovis* and *P soroptes cuniculi*), goats (*Psoroptes caprae* and *Psoroptes cuniculi*), horses (*Psoroptes equi, Psoroptes natalensis, Psoroptes ovis,* and *Psoroptes cuniculi*), and rabbits (*Psoroptes cuniculi*). It is considered to be less host specific as compared to other ectoparasites. It is most commonly seen in western, southwestern, and central United States but is rare in other parts of North America. Transmission occurs by direct and indirect contact with disease occurring more commonly during the winter months. Psoroptic mange is sometimes referred to as "body mange" in cattle, "sheep scab" in sheep, and "ear canker" in rabbits. Psoroptic mange or "scab" is reportable in cattle, sheep, and horses.
  - The mite is round, 0.4–0.8 mm in length with long legs and long three-segmented pedicels. The mite is nonburrowing and pierces the skin with its stylet-like chelicerae in order to consume serum. This is what creates the clinical lesion of a crust, hence the common name "sheep scab." Mites are primarily located on the shoulders and rump of the host, with the exception of rabbits where it is found in the ear. The life cycle on the host is completed in about 10 days, and it can live off the host in organic debris for up to 18 days in most situations. However, *P. ovis* and *P. cuniculi* can live off of the host for 48 and 84 days, respectively, in ideal environmental conditions.
  - Clinical signs include pruritus, alopecia, tail and mane seborrhea, papules, crusts, excoriations, and tail rubbing. Animals infested with *P. cuniculi* may show signs of otitis externa including head shaking, ear scratching, head shyness, and secondary bacterial/fungal infections. Lesions (thick crusts) can spread to the face and neck in severe cases. This disease creates significant damage to wool in sheep with a subsequent loss of production for farmers. Some animals may be asymptomatic.

- *Otodectes* sp. (Figure 6.40)
  - This mite belongs to the family Psoroptidae. It also is referred to as the ear mite. It affects primarily dogs and cats (*Otodectes cynotis*), but it may also

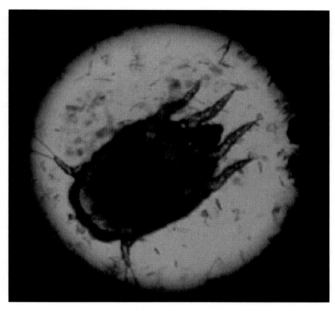

Figure 6.40 *Otodectes cynotis* ear mite from a cat. Ceruminous material was collected from the ear and rolled gently into a small amount of mineral oil on a glass slide. Then, a coverslip was applied and the slide observed under the microscope at low power (10×).

infest foxes and ferrets. It is highly contagious and is transmitted by direct or indirect contact.
- It does not burrow but lives primarily on the surface skin of the ear canal; however, it may be found anywhere on the body. The adult mite is round and has short, unsegmented pedicels with suckers on the first and second pairs of legs of the female and all legs of the male. Mites have a terminal anus. The adult appears white and can be visualized with magnification within the ear canal. The life cycle takes about 3 weeks to complete, but mites have about a 2-month life span. Mites can survive off of the host for 5–17 days in optimal conditions.
- Clinical signs are usually located to the ears and include intense pruritus and irritation with copious dark ceruminous exudate. Animals also display head shaking, ear scratching/rubbing, alopecia, aural hematoma formation, excoriations, and secondary bacterial/fungal infections. Lesions may also be found on the extremities or other places where the animal is grooming (e.g., neck, rump, and tail).
- *Cheyletiella* spp. (Figure 6.41)
  - This is a prostigmatid, nonburrowing mite with many hosts including dogs, cats, rabbits, and humans. If is commonly referred to as "walking dandruff" and infection occurs via direct and indirect contact. Mites are highly contagious, especially between young animals. *Cheyletiella yasguri* typically affects dogs, *Cheyletiella blakei* affects cats, and *Cheyletiella parasitivorax* affects rabbits. However, host specificity may not be extremely important as

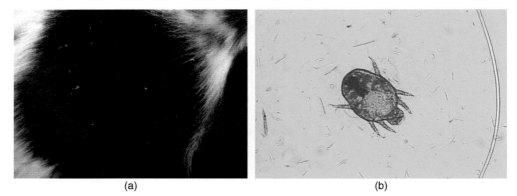

(a)   (b)

Figure 6.41   (a) *Cheyletiella parasitivorax* adult mite collected from "walking dandruff" on the dorsum of a rabbit. Scales appear as white, thin material on the surface of the hairs of the rabbit. (b) Notice the large palpal claws on the head of the adult mite at low power (10×).

Cheyletiella yasguri has been shown to affect dogs and rabbits experimentally. Humans can be transiently affected by all species of mite.

- Mites have a very characteristic appearance and can be recognized by their large saddle-shaped bodies, large palpal claws, M-shaped gnathosomal peritremes, and comb-like tarsal appendages. On the appendages are sensory organs that further aid in distinguishing between species. Specifically, the sensory organ on the first appendage is considered heart shaped in *C. yasguri*, conical shaped in *C. blakei*, and globoid shaped in *C. parasitivorax*. Mites can live for over 10 days off of the host.
- Clinical signs usually include a very mild dermatitis with excessive seborrhea (scale) on the dorsum of the host, but other signs may include variable pruritus, papules, crusts, alopecia, and excoriations. Some animals may be asymptomatic.
- Eutrombicula
  - This is a prostigmatid, nonburrowing mite with many hosts including dogs, cats, rabbits, cows, sheep, goats, horses, chickens, and humans. These mites are commonly called "chiggers." The most common species include *Eutrombicula alfreddugesi* and *Neotrombicula autumnalis*. In addition, *Walchia americana* has been reported in squirrels, rodents, and cats.
  - It is important to note that only the *larvae* are considered parasitic while the nymphs and adults are free living and nonparasitic. The larvae have six legs and a bright red to orange scutum. Infestation is usually acquired when animals are walking through brush or tall grass infested with the mites. The mite attaches to the host via formation of a stylostome through which it injects saliva to dissolve host tissue into a serious material that can be consumed easily. Mites typically remain on the host for several days for feeding unless they are dislodged by the host scratching. Chiggers are seen commonly on the concave pinna but may be anywhere on the body attached firmly to the skin.

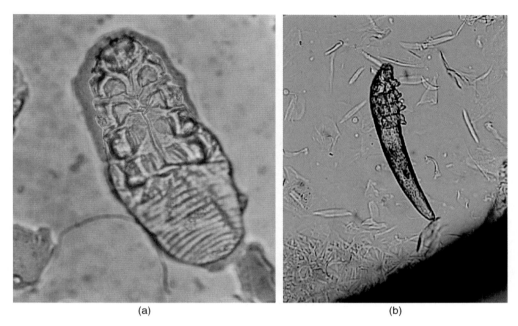

(a)   (b)

Figure 6.42   (a) This is the short bodied mite of the cat, *Demodex gatoi*. Notice that the adult mite has four pairs of legs with breast plates (10×). (b) This is the medium-bodied mite of the dog, *Demodex canis*. The mite pictured on the left was collected via deep skin scraping. The mites pictured on the right were collected via trichogram from an area of papules, crusts, and alopecia. Note that the best place to look for mites on a trichogram slide is at the hair follicle base because the mites reside deep in the follicular epithelium (10×).

- Clinical signs include intense pruritus, excoriations, alopecia, and papules. Secondary bacterial and fungal infections may occur. Pruritus may continue for days after the mite has detached. There are rare reports of paresis or chronic, painful, generalized dermatitis in dogs due to chiggers.
- Cat fur mites
  - *Lynxacarus radovsky* is the cat fur mite or the hair-clasping mite.
  - They attach themselves to the external hair shaft and are found near the top line of the cat. They cause the cat to have a scruffy appearance. Hairs have been described to have a "salt and pepper" appearance microscopically at the sites of mite attachment.
- Deep follicular mites
  - *Demodex* spp. (Figure 6.42)
    - Disease caused by these mites is referred to as red mange, follicular mange, or demodectic mange.
    - Demodex mites are considered normal flora mites in mammals and are highly species specific. They are found in the hair follicles of sebaceous glands and feed off of epithelial cells and sebum.
    - Adult demodex mites vary in body length from short-bodied to long-bodied. However, all life stages (egg, larva, nymph, and adult) are found in the diseased skin of animals. Eggs are fusiform shaped and hatch into six-legged

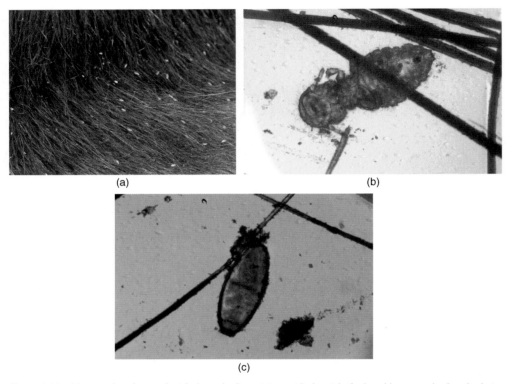

(a)   (b)

(c)

Figure 6.43   Lice can be observed with the naked eye (a) or with the aid of a hand lens attached to the hairs of the coat of this fox. Upon microscopic examination, (b) the adult louse has a broad head indicated that it is a chewing louse. (c) The eggs (nits) are observed attached to hairs upon microscopic examination (10×).

larva that molt into eight-legged nymphs and then into eight-legged adults. Adults measure 40 × 250 µm for males and 40 × 300 µm for females.

- Direct transmission occurs during nursing from the mother to the neonate during the first few days of lie.
- Clinical signs include alopecia, papules, pustules, crusts, erosions, nodules, and rarely pruritus. Lesions are usually located on the face, feet/distal extremities, or dorsal back; however, they may be present anywhere on the body. Lesions are single or multiple.
- Disease typically occurs in immune-compromised animals (e.g., young, old, or diseased patients). Identifying an underlying cause of immune suppression is required in order to adequately treat this disease.

B. Lice (Figure 6.43)
- Lice are generally classified as either chewing/biting (order Mallophaga) or sucking (order Anoplura). Lice affect numerous animals including dogs, cats, cows, small ruminants, horses, pigs, exotic animals, birds, and humans; however, they are highly host specific. Disease caused by lice is called pediculosis.
- These parasites are small, dorsoventrally flattened, wingless insects. Eggs (nits) are deposited on the host and hatch out into immature adults (nymphs). These

molt through several stages before becoming adult lice. The entire life cycle takes
several weeks (14–21 days). Lice are dependent on their host and can only
survive for a few days off of the host.
- Sucking lice are characterized by piercing mouthparts with three stylets and a
  narrow head. They have distinct pincher-like tarsal claws that aid in attaching to
  hosts. These lice feed on host blood. Lice belonging to this order include
  Linognathus spp., *Haematopinus* spp, *Polyplax* spp., and *Pediculus* spp.
- Chewing lice are characterized by stout mandibles and a broad head. All bird
  lice are chewing lice. These lice ingest a variety of epidermal materials including
  skin, hair, feathers, and sebum. Lice belonging to this order include *Damalinia*
  spp., *Trichodectes* spp., *Gliricola* spp., *Gyropus* spp, and *Felicola subrostratus*.
- Lice are well adapted to their hosts and rarely are a significant cause of mortality.
  More often, they are more of a nuisance. Lice are spread readily through direct
  and indirect contact. Crowding of animals results in rapid spread of lice between
  animals. Lice are not commonly seen in dogs and cats due to the common use of
  flea preventatives; however, stray animals may be infested with lice.
- When animals are heavily infested, sucking lice can cause anemia and weakness
  in the host. Sucking and chewing lice can cause host irritation, pruritus, papules,
  crusts, scaling, miliary dermatitis, and alopecia. Some animals may be
  asymptomatic.
C. Fleas
- These are small, brown, wingless insect with laterally compressed bodies. There
  are over 2000 species of fleas, and some fleas may affect multiple species of
  animals. The most common flea in dogs and cats is the cat flea, *Ctenocephalides
  felis felis*; however, other fleas affecting dogs and cats include *Ctenocephalides
  canis*, *Pulex* spp. (the human flea), and *Echidnophaga gallinacea* (the sticktight
  poultry flea). Similarly, fleas may affect small mammals (e.g., rabbits and ferrets)
  that are co-housed with dogs and cats. Fleas can also affect pigs, rodents, birds,
  and humans.
- *Ctenocphalides* spp. fleas have both genal and pronotal combs that distinguish
  them from other types of fleas. The rabbit flea, *Cediopsylla* sp., resembles *C.
  felis* and is distinguished by the angle of the genal teeth.
- Eggs are deposited by the adult onto the host and fall off into the environment
  where they hatch out as larvae, molt through three larval stages and one pupal
  stage, and eventually mature into the adult flea. In optimal conditions, the entire
  life cycle takes 3–4 weeks; however, it can last up to 174 days in specific
  situations. Fleas do require specific environmental conditions for optimal
  reproduction including temperatures between 20–30°C and a relative humidity
  of 70%. Adult fleas feed within minutes of acquiring a host, and females begin
  producing eggs after the very first blood meal. One adult female can produce
  40–50 eggs per day and up to 20,000 preadult forms within 2 months.
- Clinical signs caused by fleas may include papules, pustules, crusts, miliary
  dermatitis, pruritus, and alopecia. Some animals are asymptomatic.
- Fleas may also cause significant anemia and weakness in some animals,
  especially in those that are heavily infested.

- Fleas can also transmit infectious diseases such as tapeworms, rickettsial diseases, plague, bartonellosis, hemoplasma, rabbit myxomatosis virus, feline parvovirus, and leishmaniasis.

Further Reading

Ballweber, L.R. (2006) Diagnostic methods for parasitic infections in livestock. *Veterinary Clinics of North America*, 22, 695–706.

Blagburn, B. (2010) *Internal Parasites in Dogs and Cats*. Novartis Animal Health.

Bowman, D.D. (2009) *Georgis' Parasitology for Veterinarian*, (9th edn.) Saunders/Elsevier, St. Louis, MO.

Broussard, J.D. (2003) Optimal fecal assessment. *Clinical Techniques in Small Animal Practice*, 18 (4), 218–230.

De Santis, A.C., Raghavan, M., Caldanaro, J. *et al.* (2006) Estimated prevalence of nematode parasitism among pet cats in the United States. *Journal of the American Veterinary Medical Association*, 228 (6), 885–892.

Egwang, T.G. & Slocombe, J.O.D. (1982) Evaluation of the Cornell-Wisconsin centrifugation floatation technique for recovering trichostrongylid eggs from bovine feces. *Canadian Journal of Comparative Medicine*, 46, 133–137.

Foreyt, W.J. (1989) Diagnostic parasitology. *Veterinary Clinics of North America Small Animal Practice*, 19 (5), 979–1000.

Jackson, H. & Marsella, R. (2012) *BSAVA Manual of Canine and Feline Dermatology*, (3rd edn.) British Small Animal Veterinary Association, Quedgeley, Gloucester.

Katariri, S. & Oliveira-Sequeira, T.C. (2010) Comparison of three concentration methods for the recovery of canine intestinal parasites from stool samples. *Experimental Parasitology*, 126 (2), 214–216.

Kirkpatrick, C.E. (1987) Giardiasis. *Veterinary Clinics of North America Small Animal Practice*, 17 (6), 1377–1387.

Knottenbelt, D.C. (2009) *Pascoe's Principles & Practice of Equine Dermatology*, (2nd edn.) Saunders/Elsevier, St. Louis, MO.

Lee, A.C., Schantz, P.M., Kazacos, K.R. *et al.* (2010) Epidemiologic and zoonotic aspects of ascarid infections in dogs and cats. *Trends in Parasitology*, 26 (4), 155–161.

Miller, W.H., Griffin, C.E. & Campbell, K.L. (2013) *Muller & Kirk's Small Animal Dermatology*, (7th edn.) Elsevier, St. Louis, MO.

Overgaauw, P.A. & van Knapen, F. (2013) Veterinary and public health aspects of *Toxocara spp*. *Veterinary Parasitology*, 193 (4), 398–403.

Parsons, J.C. (1987) Ascarid infections of cats and dogs. *Veterinary Clinics of North America Small Animal Practice*, 17 (6), 1307–1339.

Scott, D.W. & Miller, W.H. (2003) *Equine Dermatology*. Saunders/Elsevier, St. Louis, MO.

Scott, D.W. (2007) *Color Atlas of Farm Animal Dermatology*. Blackwell Publishing Professional, Ames, Iowa.

Zajac, A.M. & Conboy, G.A. (2012) *Veterinary Clinical Parasitology*, (8th edn.) Wiley-Blackwell, Ames, IA.

Activities

Multiple Choice Questions

1. A _____ is an individual who is infested but has no symptoms of disease.
   A) Definitive host
   B) Carrier
   C) Facultative parasite
   D) Vector

2. A Hook worm is a:
   A) Protozoa
   B) Tapeworm
   C) Flat worm
   D) Round worm

3. Which is an indirect effect of a parasite on the host?
   A) Allergic response

B) Destruction of tissues
   C) Production of toxins
   D) Inhibition of host tissue growth

4. A fecal direct smear is used to identify:
   A) Coccidia
   B) Giardia
   C) Hookworm ova
   D) *Dirofilaria immitis*

5. How is *Dirofilaria immitis* transmitted?
   A) Tick
   B) Mosquito
   C) Fecal-oral
   D) Transplacental

Minimizing Laboratory Errors in Veterinary Practice

Bente Flatland
University of Tennessee, Knoxville, TN, USA

Learning Objectives

1. Understand and be able to list considerations for having an in-clinic laboratory and for using a reference laboratory.
2. Name and be able to explain the different types of laboratory error. Be able to give examples of each.
3. Be able to define *quality assurance* (QA) and *quality control* (QC).
4. Understand principles of how to minimize laboratory error. Be able to give specific examples of procedures that minimize each type of laboratory error.
5. Be able to define the term *standard operating procedure* (SOP). List advantages of SOP use.
6. Be able to define the term *quality control material* (QCM). Understand what information is provided for an assayed QCM.
7. Be able to define these terms: *running controls, control data,* and *control limits.* Be able to list three methods of interpreting control data as acceptable or unacceptable. Broadly, be able to list advantages and limitations of each method.
8. Give the traditional recommendation for how often controls should be run (i.e., how often QCM should be analyzed). Understand how this recommendation was derived and why it may differ for point-of-care testing (POCT).
9. Be able to define the term *analytical quality requirement.* List how quality requirements may be derived. Understand how quality requirements may be used.
10. Be able to define these terms: *control rule, statistical QC,* and *QC validation.* Understand what information and resources are required to perform QC validation, such that validated control rules may be used (i.e., such that statistical QC may be done).

KEY TERMS

Analytical error
Bias
Control limits
Control material
Imprecision
Preanalytical error
Postanalytical error
Quality assurance
Quality control

Clinical Pathology and Laboratory Techniques for Veterinary Technicians, First Edition.
Edited by Anne Barger and Amy MacNeill.
© 2015 John Wiley & Sons, Inc. Published 2015 by John Wiley & Sons, Inc.
Companion Website: www.wiley.com/go/barger/vettechclinpath

Introduction

Basing medical decisions on accurate laboratory data facilitates good patient care and minimizes liability. Although laboratory instruments marketed to veterinary clinics are designed for ease of use and minimal maintenance, it is important to realize that good quality data do not occur spontaneously but rather are the result of a systematic and comprehensive *quality assurance* and *quality control* (QA/QC) program. In contrast to human medicine, veterinary diagnostic laboratory testing (in any setting) is not subject to federal regulatory oversight; it is thus essential that veterinarians and veterinary technicians make a commitment to QA/QC from within the profession.

Laboratory Considerations

A. There are considerations to having an in-clinic laboratory versus using a referral laboratory. Potential benefits and limitations of having in-clinic laboratory equipment are presented in Table 7.1. Each veterinary practice must weigh the pros and cons of owning and maintaining laboratory equipment for their particular circumstances and patient population.
- General considerations include the following:
  - Time costs
  - Resource availability (e.g., space, personnel, and training)
  - Financial costs
  - Nature of the patient population served
B. Many modern veterinary practices perform a combination of in-clinic and reference laboratory testing. Reference laboratories should be selected carefully.
- General considerations for reference laboratory selection include the following:
  - Available test menu
  - Cost of testing
  - Data reporting
  - Customer service
  - Qualifications of laboratory staff (e.g., are clinical pathologists board certified? are staff certified medical technologists?)
  - Quality assurance practices
- Some reference laboratories may participate in voluntary laboratory accreditation programs.
C. If the decision is made to own and maintain in-clinic laboratory equipment, a formalized approach in which the in-clinic laboratory is considered a discrete unit within the veterinary hospital is strongly recommended.
- General laboratory functional areas are depicted in Figure 7.1.
- The in-clinic laboratory should have its own quality plan, chain-of-command, and dedicated budget.
  - The budget should include cost of the following:

Table 7.1   Considerations for in-clinic and reference laboratory testing.

Potential Benefits	Potential Limitations
Owning and maintaining in-clinic laboratory equipment	
Easy access to laboratory instruments and data	Requires a commitment to continual quality management
Analysis of fresh samples	Requires dedicated budget for maintaining instruments, reagents, control materials, laboratory supplies, and training and continuing education for staff
Rapid turn-around time for results	Requires dedicated personnel who are appropriately trained
Revenue stream	Requires time (writing and maintaining SOP's, running controls and samples, interpreting and archiving control data, performing maintenance, stocking supplies, etc.)
Can be enjoyable (e.g., if the veterinarian or veterinary technician enjoys microscopy)	Requires appropriate physical space for instrumentation and storage conditions and space for reagents, controls, and supplies
	Requires training about and appropriate handling and disposal of biological materials (including handling of potentially infectious materials)
Submitting samples to a reference laboratory	
All the practice must do is submit the correct type of sample	Longer turn-around time for results
Samples are theoretically measured, interpreted, and reported by board-certified medical technologists and clinical pathologists with training in laboratory quality management	Delay in sample handling may be an issue for certain types of tests
It may be more cost effective (on a per sample basis) than owning and maintaining in-clinic equipment	If the reference laboratory does not provide courier service, someone must deliver or ship the samples to the laboratory

- New instrument purchases
- Instrument service visits by the manufacturer (or service contracts, if applicable)
- QA services (e.g., by instrument manufacturer or independent QA consultant)
- Instrument depreciation and replacement
- Instrument reagents
- *Quality control materials* (QCMs)

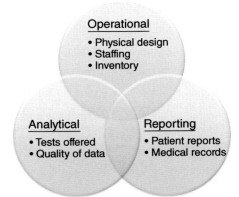

Figure 7.1 Major functional areas of a diagnostic laboratory. Each functional area should be considered in the facility's laboratory policies and quality plan.

- - Other supplies and ancillary equipment
  - Continuing education for staff engaged in laboratory testing
- The laboratory manager should be familiar with patient caseload and testing volumes, such that supplies purchased match laboratory needs and unneeded inventory does not accumulate and expire.
- In large facilities (e.g., multi-service specialty hospitals or hospitals having multiple sites), consideration should be given to the formation of a point-of-care testing (POCT) committee or working group having representation from all major POCT stakeholders in the facility.
  - Suggested composition of a POCT committee is given in Table 7.2.
  - The most likely role of a POCT committee in a veterinary hospital is as an advisory body to the various hospital services and administration regarding POCT equipment purchase, maintenance, and QA/QC.
  - In human medicine, where laboratory testing is subject to governmental oversight, POCT committees may additionally have a policing and enforcement role to ensure that various hospital testing sites comply with applicable regulations. The latter does not apply to veterinary medicine at this time, and each veterinary facility is free to decide whether its POCT committee additionally has any policing role.

Laboratory Area

A. Each veterinary facility should ensure that the area housing the in-clinic laboratory is appropriate regarding space, ambient temperature, humidity, ventilation, lighting, and water and electrical sources. Many laboratory instruments are sensitive to vibration and fluctuations in temperature, and these should be minimized.

Table 7.2   Suggested minimum composition of a veterinary POCT committee.

Perspective Represented	Rationale
Hospital or laboratory manager	Represent the facility's administrative perspective
Veterinarian(s)	Represent doctor's perspective; very large hospitals may consider having one doctor from each service represented
Veterinary technician(s)	Represent POCT operator's perspective; very large hospitals may consider having one technician from each service represented
Medical records	Help address issues concerning recording and archiving of patient data
Information technology/computer services	Facilitate interface between POCT devices and the hospital information system (electronic medical record)
Accounts/billing	Help address issues concerning the capturing and billing of POCT
External or internal QA/QC consultant	If applicable, to make recommendations concerning QA/QC procedures used

B. The laboratory area should be organized to promote efficient work flow. Appropriate consideration should be given to health and safety of laboratory staff, and work areas should be ergonomic and easy to clean and disinfect. Spill kits and wash stations should be provided as needed or required by law. Biological hazards should be appropriately handled and disposed of, and all applicable governmental regulations should be followed.

Types of Laboratory Error

Laboratory error is divided according to the phases of testing, that is, *preanalytical, analytical, and postanalytical.*

A. *Preanalytical error* occurs before the laboratory test is performed and refers to problems or variables involving sample collection, identification, and processing. Examples of preanalytical error include improper
   - Patient preparation (e.g., lack of fasting)
   - Sample container type
   - Sample storage
   - Lipemia, hemolysis, and icterus are additional preanalytical patient variables that may impact accuracy of sample analysis. Hemolysis may be either an inherent patient variable or result from improper sample handling.
B. *Analytical error* occurs while the laboratory test is being performed and may involve the instrument itself, reagents, or the instrument operator. Examples of

analytical error include blocked instrument tubing, expiring instrument lamp, inexperienced instrument operator, and use of expired reagents.
- Analytical error is further divided into (see glossary)
  - Random error (also known as *imprecision, repeatability,* or *reproducibility*)
  - Systematic error (also known as *bias* or *inaccuracy*)
    - In large, complex laboratory instruments, bias can be minimized or even eliminated through the process of *calibration* (adjusting how a laboratory instrument measures).
    - In contrast, POCT instruments typically cannot be calibrated by the operator and thus any inherent bias is fixed.
    - Bias is further divided into *constant bias* and *proportional bias* (see glossary).
  - All commonly used laboratory instrument have some inherent degree of random and systematic error (imprecision and bias); however, the degree of analytical error should not be so large that it interferes with the clinician's ability to interpret patient data. In other words, for a stable test system, the clinician should have confidence that changing patient results represent patient physiology and not merely instrument analytical variation.
    - If problems with the test system occur, analytical error can increase, causing erroneous patient results.
    - The purpose of QC procedures is to monitor test system performance and detect any analytical error that could yield inaccurate patient results, *ideally before patient samples are analyzed.*
C. *Postanalytical error* occurs after the laboratory test is performed and involves errors in data interpretation (e.g., use of inappropriate reference intervals), reporting, transcription, or archiving.
D. Studies in human medicine have shown that laboratory error rates in the POCT setting are higher than in reference laboratories and predominantly occur in the preanalytical and analytical phases of testing. A recent study in one human health care system (O'Kane et al.) showed that most POCT quality errors occurred in the analytical phase of testing and stemmed from operator failure to undertake basic instrument preparation and maintenance, rather than from instrument failure per se.

Minimizing Laboratory Error

Generation of accurate laboratory data requires ongoing planning for and assessment of quality. A continuous quality planning cycle is depicted in Figure 7.2. A list of recommended general QA procedures is given in Table 7.3.

Minimizing All Types of Laboratory Error

A. Use of written policies and standard operating procedures (SOPs) is strongly recommended.
- SOPs should be written for all laboratory procedures and include step-by-step instructions regarding the preanalytical, analytical, and postanalytical phases of testing.

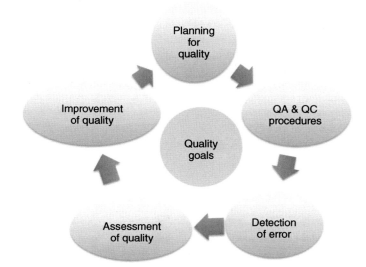

Figure 7.2   The lynchpin of the quality cycle is having specific quality goals that allow planning for quality. From there, QA/QC procedures can be implemented, monitored, and assessed, with improvements made as needed on a continual basis. When error is detected, efficacy of corrective actions should be assessed and documented.

Table 7.3   Recommended general quality assurance procedures for in-clinic veterinary laboratories.

QA Procedures	Type of Error Minimized or Eliminated
Use of written policies, standard operating procedures, and forms	All types
Adequate personnel training (initial and ongoing)	All types
Participation in an EQA (proficiency testing) program	All types
Analysis of only properly obtained and handled samples	Preanalytical
Documentation of regular instrument maintenance, repairs, and upgrades	Analytical
Proper storage and handling of reagents and QCM	Analytical
Use of medical repeat and review criteria	Analytical
Use of appropriate reference intervals	Postanalytical
Accurate transference of patient data into medical records	Postanalytical

Explanations of specific procedures are given in the text.

- One SOP per laboratory instrument or procedure is recommended. Suggestions for SOP content can be found in other resources.
- SOPs should be readily available to all staff engaged in laboratory testing.

- SOP use ensures that laboratory procedures are carried out in an accurate and consistent manner. In addition, they may be used for staff training and competency assessment.
B. Maintaining a separate instrument log for each laboratory instrument in the clinic is also strongly recommended.
  - Instrument logs may be used for documenting routine maintenance, repairs, upgrades, and occurrence/investigation/resolution of any problems; these can also be used for archiving control data (see the following text).
  - The instrument log, manufacturer-provided user manual, and SOP should be kept in close proximity to instruments such that staff can readily access them during routine operations.

TECHNICIAN TIP 7–1　The veterinary facility should have a document control policy in place, such that only current, approved copies of policies and SOPs are in circulation.

C. All personnel engaged in laboratory testing should be appropriately trained.
  - Training should be documented (e.g., in training logs or individual personnel files).
  - Provision should be made for initial training and for ongoing continuing education.
  - Periodic competency assessment of laboratory staff (e.g., by the hospital or laboratory manager) is recommended and results should be documented.
  - Staff training and education resources include the following:
    - Laboratory quality management consultants
      - Board-certified veterinary clinical pathologists
      - Certified medical technologists
      - Instrument manufacturer representatives
    - Training programs available through instrument manufacturers
    - Regional and national veterinary continuing education meetings
    - On-line resources (e.g., Veterinary Information Network [VIN, available at www.vin.com] or Westgard QC, Inc. [available at www.westgard.com])
D. Participating in an external quality assurance (EQA, also known as proficiency testing) program is strongly recommended if a suitable program is available.
  - Data provided to participants vary by EQA program provider but generally include means, standard deviations, and other statistics comparing the participating laboratory's results to a peer group using the same or similar instrumentation.
  - Quarterly participation is ideally recommended, but participation two or three times per year may be sufficient.
  - Identification of an appropriate peer group to which the participating laboratory's results can be compared is critical to successful EQA participation, and a limitation of this recommendation for in-clinic laboratories at this time is that POCT analytical methods are underrepresented in currently available veterinary EQA programs.

E. Promoting a "culture of quality" within the in-clinic laboratory is essential.
  - Staff engaged in laboratory testing should be encouraged to report and investigate possible errors.
  - Quality errors, trouble-shooting procedures, and efficacy of corrective actions should be documented in instrument logs.

> **TECHNICIAN TIP 7–2**   A chain-of-command should be specified, such that trouble shooting and resolution of quality problems are overseen by appropriately trained personnel.

Minimizing Preanalytical Error

A. Preanalytical error is an important source of error for both in-clinic and send-out (i.e., to a reference laboratory) testing. Minimizing preanalytical error requires proper following list
  - Patient preparation
    - Patients should be fasted as needed.
    - Vigorous exercise should be avoided immediately before sample collection.
  - Sample collection technique
    - Venipuncture and cystocentesis should be performed carefully by properly trained personnel and with minimal trauma, in order to minimize patient hemorrhage, sample hemolysis, and activation of clotting proteins and platelets (the latter is particularly crucial for coagulation testing).
    - Excessive excitement and stress should be minimized during sample collection.
    - Samples should be collected into containers/tubes appropriate for the tests being performed. Adequate sample volumes should be obtained; however, taking excessive blood volumes should be avoided to minimize any negative impact of sampling on patient health.
    - In the case of plasma or serum chemistry analytes, the plasma or serum should be separated from the cells in a timely manner by centrifugation and subsequent pipetting.
      - Plasma samples may be centrifuged immediately following collection.
      - Serum samples should be allowed to clot before centrifugation.

> **TECHNICIAN TIP 7–3**   Separation of plasma or serum within 30–60 minutes is a general recommendation.

  - Sample identification
    - Samples should be properly identified at the time of collection by animal name and/or identification number.
    - Sample date and time should also be recorded.
  - Sample storage
    - Samples should be kept at appropriate temperatures at all times (before, during, and after processing).
    - Light-sensitive samples should be wrapped or kept in the dark.

- Blood smears and cytologic preparations should be kept away from formalin fumes; such samples should be packaged separately from biopsy specimens if these are to be shipped to a reference laboratory.
- Samples should be analyzed as soon as possible; samples should be stored appropriately if there is to be a delay between sample acquisition and analysis.
- For send-out tests, clinic personnel should consult with the reference laboratory as needed to ensure proper sample handling during shipment.

Minimizing Analytical Error

A. Error flags
  - Should be promptly investigated when they occur.
  - Following problem correction, patient samples should be reanalyzed as needed.
  - In addition to error flags, POCT instruments or their consumable unit devices (cartridges, rotors, slides, or strips) may possess built-in, electronic (or other) QC functions that monitor analytical processes of the instrument.
    - Instrument operators should be familiar with these internal instrument QC functions, monitor any resulting data on a regular basis, and investigate problems as needed.
B. Historically, the cornerstone of laboratory QC has been analysis of liquid QCM ("running controls") and the generation of control data.
  - Archiving control data is strongly recommended. QCM lot numbers should be recorded along with control data. Archiving options include the following:
    - The instrument itself (if software has this capability)
    - An instrument log
    - A computer spreadsheet
  - Proper storage and handling of QCM is essential to good QC. Expired QCM should never be used, and the manufacturer's instructions for QCM storage and handling should be followed.
  - Liquid QCMs are designated as assayed or non-assayed. Use of assayed materials is recommended.
    - For assayed materials, the QCM manufacturer provides a known concentration range (i.e., minimum and maximum) ± other descriptive statistics (mean, standard deviation, and/or coefficient of variation) for all analytes in that QCM.
    - QCM may be available in several "levels" (ranges of analyte concentration, e.g., low, normal, and high, or normal and abnormal).
    - Commercially available QCM are human-origin materials (made from human blood products, with added preservatives and possibly added animal-source or synthetic components).

TECHNICIAN TIP 7-4   Ideally, veterinary practices should purchase assayed QCM analyzed by the same or similar analytical methods as used by their own instrument. The instrument manufacturer may also sell QCM.

- As the purpose of running controls is to screen for analytical error, out-of-control data suggest that analytical error is present and should prompt investigation of the test system (operator, instrument, and reagents).
  - Following problem correction, controls should be repeated.
  - Patient samples should only be analyzed after repeat QCM analysis demonstrates in-control (acceptable) results.
C. Traditional, optimal QC frequency is to run controls once daily, that is, once every 24 hours on each day that the instrument is to be used for patient samples. (High-volume laboratories may run controls more frequently, e.g., once per shift.)
  - This optimal recommendation stems from regulatory requirements in human medicine and is based on the principles that
    - Analysis of external QCM is the only way to monitor function of the entire analytical system (instrument, reagents, and operator).
    - Complexity of instruments traditionally used in reference laboratories is such that daily monitoring of instrument function is prudent.
  - POCT instruments are less technologically complex and designed to be relatively maintenance free.
    - In addition, many POCT instruments (particularly those used for analysis of biochemistry analytes) use consumable (disposable) unit devices such as cartridges, rotors, slides, or strips. These unit devices vary in technological sophistication and complicate QC frequency recommendations in several ways.
      - First, a unit device must be used each time controls are run, adding expense to the QC process.
      - Second, a QC run technically only evaluates quality of that one particular unit device; quality of the other unit devices within that lot is assumed.
      - And third, many POCT instruments have built-in quality functions designed to assess the instrument's electronic performance; generally, such QC functions are considered complimentary to, but not a substitute for, analysis of external liquid control samples.
  - Recommendations for QC frequency for veterinary POCT instruments are summarized in Figure 7.3.
D. Control data must be interpreted as acceptable ("in-control") or unacceptable ("out-of-control"). The *control limits* that are used to interpret control data affect the sensitivity and specificity of analytical error detection.
  - Analytical error may be thought of as "disease" within the test system.
    - Running controls is analogous to using diagnostic testing to detect disease in a patient.
    - Control limits are analogous to medical decision thresholds used to decide whether disease is present or absent (whether the test is positive or negative).
    - A given set of control limits has a certain sensitivity (known as *probability of error detection* or P_{ed}) and specificity (represented by *probability of false rejection* or P_{fr}) for detecting analytical error.
    - Ideally, control limits have both high P_{ed} and low P_{fr}; otherwise, medically important analytical error may be missed and a high rate of "false alarms" adds time and expense to the QC process.

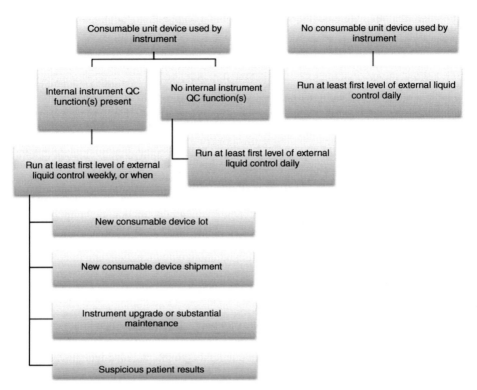

Figure 7.3   Control data should be interpreted as "in control" or "out-of-control" according to predetermined control limits (see text). Out-of-control data suggest laboratory error and should be investigated. Patient samples should not be analyzed until trouble shooting and repeat analyses of control material indicate proper test system function. Control data should be archived, such that data trends can be monitored.

- A particular instrument's analytical performance (its inherent random and systematic error) is a limiting factor in the sensitivity and specificity of given control limits for detecting analytical error.
  - For a given QCM and the same control limits used with two different instruments, one having strong analytical performance (minimal inherent error) and one having weaker performance (more inherent error), P_{ed} and P_{fr} will be better (higher and lower, respectively) for the instrument with inherently stronger analytical performance.
  - If a given P_{ed} and P_{fr} are desired, it is important to realize that given control limits may not be able to "achieve" this P_{ed} and P_{fr} if instrument analytical performance is weak.
- E. Three approaches to control data interpretation exist and not are mutually exclusive.
  - Compare control data to the manufacturer's reported range for the QCM being used (i.e., use the manufacturer's reported minimum and maximum as the control limits).

- This should always be done, as data falling outside these reported ranges likely reflect egregious error, which must be investigated and addressed.
- A limitation of this approach is that it has lower sensitivity for analytical error detection (lower P_{ed}) than other types of control limits; QCM manufacturer-reported ranges are typically based on data from numerous instruments (and even multiple laboratories) and are thus relatively wide.
- It is possible for medically important analytical error to be present in a given, individual laboratory (based on an analytical quality requirement, see the following text) and control data still to be within reported ranges.
- Ideally, QCM manufacturer-reported ranges should be used as temporary guidelines, until the laboratory or clinic establishes its own means, standard deviations, and control limits.
- An alternative approach is to plot control data over time using control charts (e.g., Levey–Jennings charts).
  - Control charts plot analyte concentration on the y-axis and time (day or run number) on the x-axis.
  - Control charts are useful for spotting individual out-of-control data points and shifts (*drift*) in data over time.
  - Traditionally, when using control charts, data points considered out-of-control (unacceptable) are those greater than ± two (or three) standard deviations (SD) away from the mean of the data, that is, control limits equal the values ± 2SD (or ± 3SD) from the mean.
  - Mean ± 2SD and mean ± 3SD can be thought of as *control rules* that determine the control limits. The rule "mean ± 2SD" (also written as 1_{2s}) has high P_{ed}; however, a limitation of this rule is that resulting control limits have higher-than-ideal P_{fr}. In other words, some data considered out-of-control based on this rule may not truly represent medically important analytical error and cause unnecessary repetition of QCM analysis or other trouble-shooting activity. Information regarding control rule nomenclature can be found in other resources.
  - Software built into some laboratory instruments automatically archives control data and creates control charts. If an instrument does not have this capability and control chart use is desired, then graphs must be created by hand or using commercially available software.
  - Representative Levey–Jennings charts are shown in Figure 7.4.
- Mean ± 2SD (1_{2s}) and mean ± 3SD (1_{3s}) are not the only rules available for determining control limits. Collectively, the various available control rules are also known as Westgard Rules. Westgard rules are most often used in statistical QC.
  - On the basis of previous research using large, simulated control data sets, performance characteristics (P_{ed} and P_{fr} and whether they predominantly detect random or systematic error) of various Westgard rules are known.
  - Statistical QC using validated control rules is the most stringent and targeted approach to control data interpretation (i.e., the approach that is most likely to result in reliable detection of medically important analytical error with a

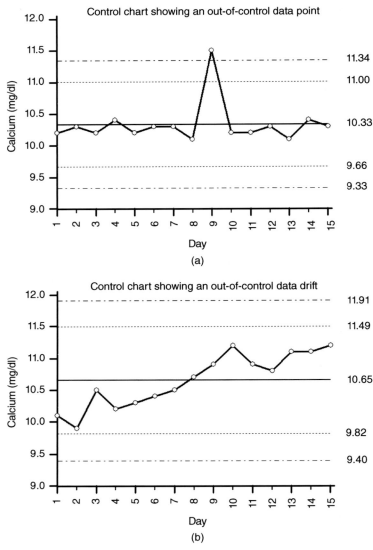

Figure 7.4 (a) The data point on Day 9 exceeds 3SD away from the mean and is unacceptable (out-of-control). Sources of error (particularly those causing increased random error) should be investigated. Examples of problems that may cause increased random error include bubbles in reagent lines, pipetting errors, unstable electrical supply, and operator errors. Lines parallel to the x-axis and numbers to the right of the graph represent mean (solid line) and ±2SD and ± 3SD (dashed lines) of the data, respectively. (b) A clear upward trend in the data is visible, and sources of error (particularly those causing increased systematic error) should be investigated. Examples of problems that may cause increased systematic error include expiring instrument lamps, deterioration of reagents, and temperature problems.[14] Lines parallel to the x-axis and numbers to the right of the graph represent mean (solid line) and ±2SD and ± 3SD (dashed lines) of the data, respectively.

low probability of false positives). QC validation requires a validation tool (e.g., calculator, table, or software) and the following information:
- A predetermined analytical quality requirement (see the following text)
- A desired P_{ed} and P_{fr}
- Data from an instrument performance study (i.e. imprecision and bias of the laboratory instrument in question).

TECHNICIAN TIP 7–5   QC validation may require collaboration with a QC consultant. QC consultations may be available through the instrument manufacturer, a private QC consultant (e.g., board-certified veterinary clinical pathologist working for a private firm or in academia), or other resources.

F. Use of an analytical quality requirement is central to the principles of QC validation and statistical QC.
- Analytical quality requirements may be based on
  - Medical decision thresholds
  - Biologic variation data
  - Governmental regulatory requirements
  - Consensus recommendations from expert bodies
- An analytical quality requirement must be chosen *for each analyte measured*. Analytical quality requirements may vary by:
  - Analyte type
  - Analyte concentration
  - Species
- The American Society for Veterinary Clinical Pathology (ASVCP) recommends use of *allowable total error* (TE_a), a type of analytical quality requirement based on medical decision thresholds and the consensus opinion of veterinary experts.
- TE_a for a given analyte can be compared to an instrument's calculated *observed total error* (TE_{obs}) for that analyte in order to determine whether instrument performance is suitable.

Minimizing Postanalytical Error

A. Numerical instrument data that are known to be inaccurate (e.g., automated platelet counts from samples having platelet clumping) should not be reported.
B. If paper medical records are used, instrument print outs should be archived in the patient medical record.
C. If data are recorded in the patient medical record manually (rather than via electronic download from the instrument to the hospital information system), a system should be in place to ensure that no transcription errors have occurred.

D. Annotations to patient laboratory data (whether on paper or electronic) should be initialed and dated.
  • Hematology data are most likely to require annotations, as blood smear review may yield morphological information that should be added to the patient report.

Summary

Although laboratory instruments and test kits marketed to veterinary clinics are designed to be easy to use and relatively maintenance-free, generation of good quality patient data nonetheless requires a comprehensive quality assurance program that seeks to minimize error in all phases of laboratory testing. Veterinary practices are encouraged to take a formalized approach to laboratory QA and QC that considers the in-clinic laboratory as a defined unit within the hospital facility having its own physical space, budget, policies, procedures, records, and personnel. Many quality errors occurring in POCT settings are preventable with adequate instrument operator training and adherence to SOPs. Veterinary technicians play a key role in this process, as they are most likely to obtain and handle patient samples and function as laboratory instrument operators.

Further Reading

Burtis, C.A., Ashwood, E.R., & Bruns, D.E. (eds.) (2006) *Tietz Textbook of Clinical Chemistry and Molecular Diagnostics* (4th ed.). Elsevier Saunders, St. Louis, MO.

Farr, A.J. & Freeman, K.P. (2010) Quality control validation, application of sigma metrics and performance comparison between two biochemistry analyzers in a commercial veterinary laboratory. *Journal of Veterinary Diagnostic Investigation*, 20, 536–544.

Flatland, B., Freeman, K.P., Friedrichs, K.R., *et al.* (2010) ASVCP quality assurance guidelines: control of general analytical factors in veterinary laboratories. *Veterinary Clinical Pathology*, 39, 264–277.

Flatland, B., Freeman, K.P., Vap, L.M., & Harr, K.E. ASVCP guidleines: quality assurance for point-of-care testing in veterinary medicine. *Veterinary Clinical Pathology* 2013; 42(4):405–423.

Flatland, B., & Vap, L.M. (2012) Quality management recommendations for automated and manual in-house hematology of domestic animals. *The Veterinary Clinics of North America Small Animal Practice*, 42, 11–22.

Freeman, K.P. & Gruenwaldt, J. (1999) Quality control validation in veterinary laboratories. *Veterinary Clinical Pathology*, 28, 150–155.

Harr, K.E, Flatland, B., Nabity, M., & Freeman, K.P. ASVCP guidelines: allowable total error guidelines for biochemistry. *Veterinary Clinical Pathology* 2013; 42(4):424–436.

Jensen, A.L., & Kjelgaard-Hansen, M. (2010) Subjectivity in defining quality specifications for quality control and test validation. *Veterinary Clinical Pathology*, 39, 133–135.

Kenny, D., Fraser, C.G., Hyltoft Petersen, P., *et al.* (1999) Consensus agreement. *Scandinavian Journal Clinical Laboratory Investigation*, 59, 585.

Lester, S., Harr, K.E., Rishniw, M., *et al.* (2013) Current quality assurance concepts and considerations for quality control of in-clinic biochemistry testing. *Journal of the American Veterinary Medical Association*, 242, 182–192.

Meier, F.A., & Jones, B.A. (2005) Point-of-care testing error: sources and amplifiers, taxonomy, prevention strategies, and detection monitors. *Archives Pathology and Laboratory Medicine*, 129, 1262–1267.

O'Kane, M.J., McManus, P., McGowan, N., *et al.* (2011) Quality error rates in point-of-care testing. *Clinical Chemistry*, 57, 1267–1271.

Price, C.P., St John, A., & Kricka, L.L. (eds). (2010) *Point-of-Care Testing Needs, Opportunity and Innovation* (3rd ed.). AACC Press, Washington, DC.

Rishniw, M., Pion, P.D., & Maher, T. (2012) The quality of veterinary in-clinic and reference laboratory biochemical testing. *Veterinary Clinical Pathology*, 41, 92–109.

Stockham, S.L., & Scott, M.A. (2008) *Fundamentals of Veterinary Clinical Pathology* (2nd ed.). Blackwell Publishing Professional, Ames, IA.

Wayne, P.A. (2007) Clinical and Laboratory Standards Institute (CLSI). Using proficiency testing to improve the clinical laboratory; approved guideline. Clinical and Laboratory Standards Institute (CLSI).

Westgard, J.O. (ed). (2010) *Basic QC Practices* (3rd ed.). Westgard QC, Madison, WI.

Westgard, J.O. (ed). (2000) *Basic Method Validation* (3rd ed.). Westgard QC, Madison, WI.

Westgard, J.O. (ed). (2000) *Basic Planning for Quality*. Westgard QC, Madison, WI.

Westgard, J.O. (2005) *EZ Rules Version 3*. Westgard QC, Madison, WI.

Wiegers, A.L. (2004) Laboratory quality considerations for veterinary practitioners. *Journal of the American Veterinary Medical Association*, 225, 1386–1390.

Activities

Multiple Choice Questions

1. Analytical error occurring in a negative direction is:
   A) Systematic error
   B) Total allowable error
   C) Random error
   D) Bias

2. Procedure that monitors or improves laboratory performance in all phases of laboratory testing.
   A) Quality assurance
   B) Quality control
   C) Point of care testing
   D) Repeat criteria

3. Which is a cause of analytical error?
   A) Improper storage
   B) Lipemia
   C) Incorrect container type
   D) Expired reagents

4. True/False. Bias can be eliminated by calibrating an instrument.

5. True/False. A reference interval can be used interchangeably between different equipment.

6. Which can be used to minimize preanalytical error?
   A) Patient samples should be reanalyzed
   B) Samples should be appropriately labeled
   C) Error flags should be evaluated
   D) Instrument QC should be performed on a regular basis

7. True/False. The purpose of running controls is to screen for analytic error.

Glossary of Terms

Acidemia – A decrease in the pH of blood. Can be caused by metabolic or respiratory diseases.

Activated clotting time (ACT) – The time required for blood to clot after the addition of particulate material. Used to evaluate intrinsic and common coagulation pathways.

Activated partial thromboplastin time (APTT or PTT) – The time required for citrated blood to clot after phospholipid, contact activators, and calcium are added to the sample. Used to evaluate intrinsic and common coagulation pathways.

Active sediment – If there is inflammation, bacteria or crystals in the urine sediment, this indicates an active sediment.

Alanine aminotransferase (ALT) – Enzyme found in hepatocytes and skeletal muscle cells, usually, is elevated in patients with hepatocellular damage.

Albumin – Most common protein in blood, providing the majority of oncotic pressure. It is produced by the liver.

Alkalemia – An increase in the pH of blood. Can be caused by metabolic or respiratory diseases.

Alkaline phosphatase (ALP) – Membranous enzyme, primarily on hepatocytes but also found on osteoblasts, intestine, placenta, and renal tubules. The primary source in animals is liver.

Amylase – An enzyme responsible for digestion of starches and other sugars, can be elevated in pancreatitis or in a dehydrated patient.

Clinical Pathology and Laboratory Techniques for Veterinary Technicians, First Edition.
Edited by Anne Barger and Amy MacNeill.
© 2015 John Wiley & Sons, Inc. Published 2015 by John Wiley & Sons, Inc.
Companion Website: www.wiley.com/go/barger/vettechclinpath

Analytical quality requirement – A benchmark to which the analytical quality of a given instrument is compared. Analytical quality requirements are used to assess instrument performance, to compare results from two difference instruments (comparability testing), and in quality control validation.

Anemia – Decreased numbers of erythrocytes in the blood as compared to a reference interval.

Anion gap – A calculation used to show the difference between unmeasured cations and unmeasured anions in the blood.

Antidiuretic hormone (ADH) – Also called vasopressin, is a hormone produced by the pituitary gland that acts on the collecting ducts and tubules to absorb water.

Antithrombin III (ATIII) – A naturally occurring protein that neutralizes thrombin and limits coagulation.

Anuria – Lack of urine production by the kidney.

Aspartate aminotransferase (AST) – Enzyme found in hepatocytes and skeletal muscle cells, usually is elevated in patients with hepatocellular damage and severe muscle damage.

Azotemia – An increase in blood urea nitrogen (BUN) or serum creatinine as the result of dehydration, elevated with renal disease or postrenal obstruction.

Bactiuria – The presence of bacteria in the urine.

Basophil – A granulocyte with acidic cytoplasmic granules that stain blue with Romanowski-type cellular dyes. This type of blood cell is infrequently observed in circulation.

Bile – Fluid produced by the liver essential for digestion.

Bile acids – A component of bile which aids in the digestion of fats. Also a diagnostic test used to evaluate liver function.

Bilirubin – An orange pigment derived from catabolism of heme that is conjugated by the liver.

Bilirubinuria – The presence of bilirubin in the urine, indicates liver disease in most species but can be normal in dogs.

Blood urea nitrogen (BUN) – Product primarily synthesized by the liver and excreted by the kidney. It is a parameter used to evaluate azotemia.

Buccal mucosal bleeding time (BMBT) – The time required for bleeding to stop after controlled puncture of the mucosa. Used to evaluate endothelial cell and platelet functions.

Carrier – An individual who is infested but has no symptoms of disease.

Cast – Casts are protein-rich structures produced in the distal renal tubule and can indicate renal tubular damage. Casts are classified by their internal structure, that is, cellular, fatty, and so on.

Centrifuge – Equipment that separates components in a sample suspension by spinning the sample using centrifugal acceleration. Larger particles in the sample sediment out at the bottom, whereas lighter particles settle at the top of the centrifuged sample.

Cholestasis – Decreased bile flow from either intrahepatic or extrahepatic causes.

Cholesterol – An important component of lipid metabolism, often increased in patients with endocrine disease such as hypothyroidism or cholestatic disease.

Citrate – A solution of sodium citrate used to prevent the formation of a blood clot (by binding calcium) and preserve whole blood samples. Preferred anticoagulant for coagulation function tests. Anticoagulant present in blue-topped blood collection tubes.

Coagulation – The interaction of damaged cells and coagulation factors that result in the formation of an insoluble fibrin clot.

Coagulation factors – Components involved in the coagulation cascade.

Complete blood count (CBC) – A clinical pathology data set that describes circulating blood cells.

Control data – Data resulting from analysis of quality control material. Control data must be interpreted as acceptable ("in-control") or unacceptable ("out-of-control"). Decision thresholds used to determine acceptability of control data are known as *control limits*. Control limits may be determined by *control rules*.

Creatine kinase (CK) – Enzyme found in muscle myocytes.

Creatinine – A nitrogenous compound formed during normal muscle metabolism and excreted by the kidney.

Cystocentesis – A method of urine collection where urine is aspirated from the bladder with needle and syringe.

D-dimer – A fragment of fibrin formed during fibrin degradation. Used to evaluate fibrinolysis.

Definitive host – The host that harbors the adult stage of the parasite.

Diabetes mellitus – Disease resulting in marked hyperglycemia either from lack of insulin or other disorder of carbohydrate metabolism.

Differential cell counter – Equipment used to track the percentage of cell subsets in a sample.

Direct life cycle – A life cycle in which a parasite is transmitted directly from one host to the next without an intermediate host or vector or another species. Contrast-indirect life cycle.

Disease – The debilitating effects of infection by a parasite (pathogen) on a host.

Disseminated intravascular coagulation (DIC) – Formation of blood clots throughout the body that leads to organ failure.

Document control policy – A policy dictating how documents used by a facility or organization are written, formatted, approved, distributed, archived, and removed from circulation, such that only current, approved document copies are available to personnel.

Electrolyte – Charged molecules are present in serum or plasma; examples include sodium, chloride, potassium, magnesium, bicarbonate, calcium, and phosphorus.

Endoparasite – A parasite that lives within the body.

Endothelial cells – Cells that line the blood vessels.

Enzyme – A catalyst of chemical reactions which does not result in degradation of the enzyme itself.

Eosinophil – A granulocyte with basic cytoplasmic granules that stain red with Romanowski-type cellular dyes. This type of blood cell is present in very low numbers in peripheral blood of healthy animals.

Erratic (or aberrant) parasite – A parasite that has entered an organ or host in which it does not ordinarily live.

Error flags – Codes or symbols displayed by laboratory instruments together with patient data when sample or analytical problems occur. Error flag meanings and triggers are explained in an instrument's user manual.

Error, random (also known as imprecision) – Analytical error occurring in either a positive or a negative direction, occurrence of which cannot be predicted.

Error, systematic (also known as inaccuracy or bias) – Analytical error occurring in one direction (a systematic shift). Systematic error may occur throughout the range of measured values (constant bias) or may be concentration-dependent (i.e., increase as analyte concentration increases or decreases, known as proportional bias).

Erythrocyte (red blood cell; RBC) – A blood cell that contains large amounts of hemoglobin which transports oxygen to and removes carbon dioxide from tissues. Mature mammalian erythrocytes do not contain a nucleus and are the most abundant blood cell type in peripheral blood.

Erythrocytosis – Increased percentage of erythrocytes in the blood as compared to a reference interval.

Ethylenediaminetetraacetic acid (EDTA) – A substance that chelates calcium, prevents blood clot formation, and preserves whole blood. Preferred anticoagulant for complete blood cell analysis. Anticoagulant is present in purple-topped blood collection tubes.

External quality assessment program (also known as proficiency testing program) – A program that evaluates a participating laboratory's total testing performance by comparing test results from that laboratory to a known standard or to an appropriate peer group mean generated from an inter-laboratory comparison in which multiple laboratories measure the same sample using the same test methods, reagents, and controls.

Facultative parasite – An organism that is capable of living either free or as a parasite.

Fibrin degradation products (FDP) – Protein fragments produced during degradation of fibrin by plasmin. Used to evaluate fibrinolysis.

Fibrinogen (Factor I) – A coagulation factor in plasma that is converted into fibrin by thrombin.

Fibrinolysis – Breakdown of a fibrin clot.

Gamma glutamyl transferase (GGT) – An enzyme found on biliary epithelial cells.

Globulins – A family of proteins that include immunoglobulins.

Glomerular filtration rate (GFR) – The rate at which substances, such as creatinine, are filtered through the glomeruli of the kidney.

Glomerulus – Component of the nephron that consists of a tuft of capillaries.

Hematocrit (Hct) – The percentage of erythrocytes in a peripheral whole blood sample.

Hematuria – The presence of red blood cells in the urine.

Hemoconcentration – Decreased fluid volume in the blood.

Hemocytometer – A chamber used to count cells in solution. The chamber is examined microscopically, cells are counted in a structured way, and a calculation is used to determine the number of cells per microliter in a sample.

Hemoglobin concentration (Hb or Hgb) – The amount of hemoglobin is present in a whole blood sample. Vitally important for oxygen delivery to tissues. Often measured in grams/deciliter (g/dL).

Hemoglobinuria – The presence of hemoglobin in the urine.

Hemolytic index – The level of hemolysis found in plasma or serum.

Hemostasis – The cessation of bleeding involving vasoconstriction and the coagulation cascade.

Heparin – A sulfated glycosaminoglycan that potentiates antithrombin III functions, prevents blood clot formation, and preserves whole blood. Anticoagulant present in green-topped blood collection tubes.

Hepatic – Referring to the liver.

Hepatic lipidosis – A metabolic disease resulting in lipid deposition in the hepatocytes.

Hepatitis – Inflammation of the liver.

Hepatocytes – Predominant cell type of the liver.

Host – An organism that harbors a parasite.

Hyper- – A prefix used to indicate an increase in a laboratory value, for example, hyperbilirubinemia, indicates an elevated bilirubin in the blood.

Hyperadrenocorticism(Cushing's disease) – An endocrine disease resulting in excessive production of cortisol.

Hypertonic – A fluid that has more solute than another fluid.

Hypo- – A prefix used to indicate a decrease in a laboratory value, for example, hypokalemia, indicates a decreased potassium level in the blood.

Hypoadrenocorticism (Addison's disease) – A disease affecting the adrenal cortex resulting in a decrease in cortisol and/or mineralocorticoids.

Hyposthenuria – Urine-specific gravity <1.008, indicates active dilution of urine by the kidneys.

Hypotonic – A fluid that has less solute than another fluid.

Icteric – A yellow coloring of the patient or plasma resulting from an elevated bilirubin.

Indirect life cycle – A life cycle that requires one or more intermediate hosts before the definitive host species is reinfected. Contrast with direct life cycle.

Infection – Occurrence of parasites in a host (which is not necessarily manifested by disease). A host is infected by endoparasites.

Infestation – Occurrence of parasites on a host (which is not necessarily manifested in disease). A host is infested by ectoparasites.

Interleukin – A chemical mediator that affects cellular development and function. Involved in hematopoiesis, immunologic reactions, cell signaling, cell cycling, and many other bodily functions.

Intermediate host – The host that harbors the larval stages of the parasite.

Isosthenuria – Urine-specific gravity of 1.008–1.012, indicating that the kidney is not concentrating or diluting the urine.

Lactate dehydrogenase (LDH) – A cytosolic enzyme of muscle.

Leukocyte (white blood cell; WBC) – Blood cells involved in immune functions including granulocytes, lymphocytes, and monocytes.

Leukocytosis – Increased numbers of leukocytes in the blood as compared to a reference interval.

Leukopenia – Decreased numbers of leukocytes in the blood as compared to a reference interval.

Lipase – A pancreatic enzyme which is often elevated in patients with pancreatitis.

Lipemia – An increased amount of triglyceride carrying lipoproteins in the blood resulting in a milky appearance to plasma or serum.

Lymphocyte – A leukocyte that is critical for development of adaptive immune responses. Subsets of lymphocytes include B-cells and T-cells. This type of blood cell is present in moderate numbers in peripheral blood of healthy animals.

Mean cell hemoglobin (MCH) – The average amount of hemoglobin is present within an erythrocyte. Often measured in picograms (pg).

Mean cell hemoglobin concentration (MCHC) – The average amount of hemoglobin present within an erythrocyte corrected for the volume of the erythrocyte. Often measured in grams/deciliter.

Mean cell volume or mean corpuscular volume (MCV) – The average size of an erythrocyte. Often measured in femtoliters (fL).

Mean platelet volume (MPV) – The average size of a platelet. Often measured in femtoliters.

Metamyelocyte – A hematopoietic precursor cell that develops into a granulocyte (neutrophil, eosinophil, or basophil).

Metarubricyte (nucleated red blood cell) – A hematopoietic precursor cell that develops into an erythrocyte.

Microscope – An instrument used to magnify a biological sample that is a few cell layers thick.

Monocyte – A leukocyte that becomes activated as it exits the peripheral blood and presents antigens to other cells of the immune system. This blood cell type is present in low numbers in peripheral blood of healthy mammals.

Morbidity – State of ill-health produced by a disease.

Myelocyte – A hematopoietic precursor cell that develops into a metamyelocyte.

Myoglobinuria – The presence of myoglobin pigment from muscle in urine. Its presence is indicative of severe muscle disease.

Neutrophil – A granulocyte with neutral cytoplasmic granules that do not stain with Romanowski-type cellular dyes. Segmented neutrophils are fully mature neutrophils that have a segmented nucleus and are the most abundant leukocyte in the peripheral blood of healthy cats, dogs, and horses. Band neutrophils are slightly immature neutrophils that have a horseshoe-shaped nucleus and are found in very low numbers (if at all) in the peripheral blood of healthy animals.

Nucleated red blood cell (nRBC; metarubricyte) – Immature erythrocytes that contain a condensed nucleus.

Obligatory parasite – An organism that must live a parasitic existence.

Oliguria – It is a measure of concentration of a fluid and is measured in osmoles/L. It can be used similarly to specific gravity as a method to determine the concentration of urine.

Packed cell volume (PCV) – The percentage of cells in a peripheral whole blood sample.

Parasitism – An intimate association between two specifically distinct organisms in which one benefits and one loses. The parasite is dependent on its host for at least one essential metabolic substance.

Plasma – Fluid component of blood from unclotted blood.

Platelet (thrombocyte) – A blood cell type that is critical for hemostasis. In mammals, platelets are cytoplasmic fragments that lack a nucleus and are present in significant numbers in peripheral blood of healthy animals.

Platelet count – The number of platelets per microliter of whole blood.

Point-of-care test(s) or testing (POCT) – Laboratory testing performed outside the traditional clinical pathology laboratory, often in close proximity to patients and performed by individuals having little or no formal training in laboratory quality management. POCT instruments and test kits are designed to be easy to use and relatively maintenance free.

Polychromasia – The term for cells that stain with both basophilic and eosinophilic dyes. Observed in immature RBCs called reticulocytes that stain a bluish-red color with Romanowski-type cytologic stains.

Polycythemia – Increased numbers of erythrocytes in the peripheral blood caused by increased erythropoiesis.

Polyuria – Increased urine volume. Can be associated with many different diseases including renal disease.

Postprandial – After a meal.

Pre-prandial – Before a meal, often after a fast.

Proteinuria – The presence of protein in the urine. In a patient with dilute urine and an inactive sediment, may be an early indicator of renal disease.

Prothrombin time (PT) – The time required for citrated blood to clot after thromboplastin and calcium are added to the sample. Used to evaluate extrinsic and common coagulation pathways.

Pseudoparasite – An object that is mistaken for a parasite.

Pyuria – The presence of white blood cells in the urine.

Quality assurance (QA) – Procedures that monitor and improve laboratory performance in all phases of laboratory testing (preanalytical, analytical, and postanalytical). QA procedures include planning for quality, implementation of quality procedures, monitoring and assessment of quality, and correction of quality problems.

Quality control (QC) – Procedures that monitor analytical performance of laboratory instruments and detect analytical error. QC typically refers to use of quality control materials and analysis of resulting control data. *Statistical QC* refers to the process of using validated control rules to determine control limits.

Quality control material (QCM) – A material intended by its manufacturer to be used for the quality control of laboratory testing. QCM is designed to mimic patient samples and approximate medically important analyte concentrations. Most commercially available QCM are derived from human materials.

Quality control validation – The process of choosing control rules based on known instrument analytical performance and a predetermined analytical quality requirement. See also *control data*.

Red cell distribution width (RDW) – Indication of the variation in the mean cell volume of erythrocytes in a blood sample. Reported as a percentage.

Refractometer – An instrument that measures the refractive index of a solution and converts it into a measurement of the amount of solids in the sample. For example, the refractive index of protein concentration in a fluid is converted into grams of protein per deciliter of fluid.

Repeat criteria – Criteria that establish when a laboratory test should be repeated. For example, "repeat any blood glucose having a value <40 mg/dL."

Review criteria – Criteria that establish when an individual with greater expertise should review a laboratory result. For example, "any CBC having >30,000 WBC/µL should be reviewed by a veterinarian" or "any CBC showing abnormal cells should be sent to a reference laboratory for pathologist review."

Rubriblast – A hematopoietic precursor cell that develops into a rubricyte.

Rubricyte – A hematopoietic precursor cell that develops into a metarubricyte (nRBC).

Serum – Fluid component of blood after it has clotted.

Serum iron (SI) concentration – An estimate of the amount of circulating iron in the body. This test does not detect iron stores.

Sorbitol dehydrogenase (SDH) – Cytosolic enzyme in hepatocytes is often elevated with liver disease, found primarily in horses and cattle.

Standard operating procedure (SOP) – A written document that lists considerations and detailed instructions for preanalytical, analytical, and postanalytical phases of testing for a given laboratory instrument or test procedure.

Thrombin clotting time (TCT) – The time required for citrated blood to clot after thrombin is added to the sample. Used to evaluate the common coagulation pathway.

Thrombocytopenia – Decreased numbers of platelets in the peripheral blood as compared to a reference interval.

Thrombocytopenia – A decreased number of platelets per microliter of whole blood compared to a species-specific reference interval. It may be due to destruction, decreased production, or loss of platelets.

Thrombocytosis – Increased numbers of platelets in the peripheral blood as compared to a reference interval.

Thrombopoietin – A protein that regulates the production of platelets.

Total iron binding capacity (TIBC) – An estimate of the amount of iron lacking in the peripheral blood circulation.

Transmission – The process by which a pathogen passes from a source of infection to a new host.

Urine sediment – Refers to the solid portion of the urine. Centrifugation of the urine and removal of the supernatant is necessary to evaluate the sediment.

Vector – An organism that delivers a parasite from the environment to the host.

Index

Locators in *italic* refer to figures and diagrams
Locators in **bold** refer to glossary entries

Clinical Pathology and Laboratory Techniques for Veterinary Technicians, First Edition.
Edited by Anne Barger and Amy MacNeill.
© 2015 John Wiley & Sons, Inc. Published 2015 by John Wiley & Sons, Inc.
Companion Website: www.wiley.com/go/barger/vettechclinpath

Made in United States
Orlando, FL
22 January 2023

28783833R00155